Dietary Iron: Birth to Two Years

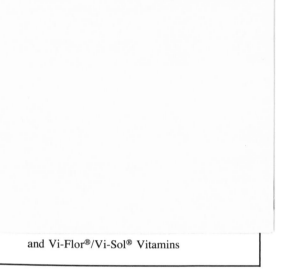

and Vi-Flor®/Vi-Sol® Vitamins

Dietary Iron:
Birth to Two Years

Editor

L. J. Filer, Jr., M.D., Ph.D.
Professor Emeritus
Department of Pediatrics
College of Medicine
University of Iowa
Iowa City, Iowa

Raven Health Care Communications

**Raven Health Care Communications, Division of Raven Press, Ltd.,
1185 Avenue of the Americas, New York, New York 10036**

Made in the United States of America

Library of Congress Cataloging-in-Publication Data

Dietary iron.

Based on the proceedings of a symposium held December 12–14, 1988
in Dallas, Tex.
Includes bibliographies and index.
1. Iron deficiency diseases in infants—Congresses. 2. Iron deficiency
diseases in children—Congresses. 3. Iron—Metabolism—Congresses. 4.
Baby foods—Iron content—Congresses. 5. Infants—Development—
Congresses. I. Filer, Lloyd J. [DNLM: 1. Anemia, Hypochromic—in
infancy & childhood—congresses. 2. Child Nutrition—congresses. 3. Infant
Nutrition—congresses. 4. Iron—metabolism—congresses.   WS 115 D565
1988]

RJ399.I75D54   1989   618.92′396   89-10378
ISBN 0-88167-571-7

Foreword

"Dietary Iron: Birth to Two Years" is the fourth symposium in the 1980s sponsored by Mead Johnson to address current issues in pediatric nutrition. We believe that the published proceedings from these symposia provide clinicians as well as research scientists involved in pediatric nutrition with comprehensive state-of-the-art publications.

In the past ten years, the incidence of childhood anemia in the U.S. has decreased in large part because of iron-fortified infant formula and cereal. Health care providers must not become complacent with this success but instead must continue all efforts to prevent iron deficiency with or without anemia. The assembled panel of experts focused in detail on the consequences of suboptimal iron intake in infants and toddlers.

We now know that a contributing factor to decreased infant stores of iron is the early introduction of cow's milk into the infant's diet. Participants discussed these findings and the role of other dietary factors on childhood iron nutrition in the U.S. and in other parts of the world.

My special thanks go to the authors for their manuscripts and discussions assembled in this book. I congratulate and thank Dr. Filer, who as editor provided extensive insight, commitment, and hard work for this symposium. It is our intent that the information exchanged and recorded in these proceedings will stimulate more study into the effects of dietary iron on the growth and development of infants and children.

George L. Baker, M.D.
Vice President and Medical Director
Mead Johnson Research Center
Bristol-Myers U.S. Nutritional Group

Acknowledgments

The symposium "Dietary Iron: Birth to Two Years" was supported by an educational grant from Mead Johnson Research Center, Evansville, Indiana. The articles presented herein represent the work and opinions of the authors and are not intended to present the opinions of the Mead Johnson Research Center or Bristol-Myers Company.

The editor wishes to thank David Irons, Patricia Cornett, and Donna Curtis for their assistance in the editing and preparation of the manuscripts for publication.

The following books have been published in the 1980s from symposia sponsored by Mead Johnson. Marcel Dekker, Inc. owns the copyright for each of the books.

Carbohydrate Intolerance in Infancy, edited by Fima Lifshitz (1982)

Vitamin and Mineral Requirements in Preterm Infants, edited by Reginald C. Tsang (1985)

Nutrition for Special Needs in Infancy: Protein Hydrolysates, edited by Fima Lifshitz (1985)

Preface

In addressing the issue of nutritional iron deficiency 20 years ago I stated, "Experience with nutritional deficiencies of sufficient magnitude to constitute public health problems has demonstrated that they can be managed through public health measures. By judicious enrichment programs involving vitamins D and C, rickets and scurvy have been eliminated as public health problems. If nutritional iron deficiency is a particular threat to the health of our infant population, should we not attempt to eliminate it by assuring an adequate iron intake in the infant dietary?" (1).

This volume, *Dietary Iron: Birth to Two Years*, details the progress made in the past two decades to understand the impact of nutritional iron deficiency during infancy on growth, psychomotor and cognitive development, work capacity and performance, and infection. These important aspects of infant growth and development had not been integrated with iron nutritional status 20 years ago; thus, the critical need for dietary iron in the early months of life was not fully appreciated. In the intervening years, the new information presented in this report has placed increased emphasis on the public health importance of providing a source or sources of dietary iron. All contributors to this volume support the thesis that the growing infant requires a dietary source of iron and that the technology exists to fortify formula and infant foods with bioavailable forms of iron.

The translation of this new information into public policy and the resultant benefits of making iron available to infants through a public assistance program such as WIC (Special Supplemental Food Program for Women, Infants and Children) are emphasized in a section describing the declining prevalence of anemia among infants and children irrespective of socioeconomic status. In the words of one of the participants, "This process can be regarded as another major model of primary prevention in child health care, similar to that of childhood immunization in the prevention and reduction of communicable disease."

Several participants concluded that infants should not be fed cow's milk during the first year of life. When cow's milk is given, it replaces iron-rich foods in the infant's diet, increases gastrointestinal blood loss, and may inhibit iron absorption. These effects reduce body iron stores and may result in iron deficiency anemia. Based upon these observations, it is prudent to prevent gastrointestinal blood loss during infancy by feeding heat-processed, iron-fortified milk or soybean formulas.

The feasibility of using stable isotopes of iron to determine iron bioavailability from infant foods is addressed. On the basis of studies reported in this volume, it was concluded that iron given as ferrous fumarate was as bioavailable as iron given as ferrous sulfate. Although considerable individual variation in iron bioavailability was noted among infants, use of stable isotopes of iron holds considerable promise for study of iron absorption from infant foods and the effects of nutrient-nutrient interaction.

The effects of iron deficiency anemia on psychomotor development during infancy is reported on the basis of two field studies, one from Chile and the other from Costa Rica. Although the studies differ somewhat in clinical design, the results are strikingly similar. On the basis of the Bayley Scale of Infant Development, both studies clearly demonstrate that iron deficiency anemia is the strongest single determinant of psychomotor performance. In both studies, it was observed that reversal of the anemic state had little discernible effect on indices of mental development or psychomotor milestones. It is unclear from these studies if these observations signify irreversible damage to the central nervous system.

In addressing the question, "Does dietary iron increase or decrease susceptibility to infection?", Walter and co-workers concluded on the basis of a literature review and clinical studies conducted in Chile that ". . . iron fortification of foods is not associated with increased susceptibility to infection; moreover, there is some evidence that an adequate iron nutrition status may be beneficial."

A report on the world nutrition situation by the United Nations in 1987 estimates that 43% of world children between birth to 4 years of age are anemic. In spite of the magnitude of this problem, there are few published studies of the influence of iron deficiency on spontaneous physical activity of children, and even fewer studies of the effect of iron deficiency on physical work capacity in children. Viteri reviews the results of work performance studies in iron-deficient and-sufficient adult humans and animals and concludes that these studies may be relevant to children until age-specific studies are undertaken.

Dallman speculates on future directions of research to promote understanding of factors important in maintaining iron homeostasis during infancy. He concludes that emphasis will be focused on regulation of absorption. This control resides within the gene that modulates transferrin receptor numbers on cell surface membranes. Understanding how iron bioavailability influences messenger RNA to regulate transferrin receptor numbers will modify future perception of iron metabolism and nutrition.

Each of the twelve chapters that comprise this volume has been prepared by an international expert. Most chapters are brief and provocative, representing the state of the art. The casual or serious reader will conclude, as I have, that the infant's need for dietary iron is of paramount importance.

L. J. Filer, Jr., M.D., Ph.D

REFERENCES

1. Filer, L. J., Jr. (1969): The USA today—is it free of public health nutrition problems? *Am. J. Public Health*, 59:327–338.

About the Editor

Dr. Filer is Professor Emeritus of Pediatrics, University of Iowa College of Medicine in Iowa City, Iowa, and Executive Director, International Life Sciences Institute/Nutrition Foundation in Washington, D.C. He is a graduate of the University of Pittsburgh (B.S., 1941; Ph.D., 1944) and of the University of Rochester School of Medicine and Dentistry (1952). During his distinguished career, Dr. Filer has provided leadership as an author, editor, lecturer, and consultant on applied and scientific issues facing the field of nutrition. Many of his 200 research publications focus on vitamin E metabolism, longitudinal studies of infant nutrition and growth, and food additives, especially aspartame. Dr. Filer is a Fellow of the American Academy of Pediatrics and the American Institute of Nutrition; a member of the American Pediatric Society, the Society for Pediatric Research, the American Society for Clinical Nutrition, and the Institute of Food Technologists; and an honorary member of the American Dietetic Association. He received the Joseph Goldberger Award in Clinical Nutrition from the American Medical Association in 1978 and the Nutrition Award from the American Academy of Pediatrics in 1988.

Contents

Contributors

Peter R. Dallman, M.D.
Department of Pediatrics
University of California at San Francisco
San Francisco, California 94143

L. J. Filer, Jr., M.D., Ph.D.
Professor Emeritus
Department of Pediatrics
College of Medicine
University of Iowa
Iowa City, Iowa 52242

Frank A. Oski, M.D.
Department of Pediatrics
John Hopkins University School of Medicine
Baltimore, Maryland 21205

George M. Owen, M.D.
Bristol-Myers International Group
New York, New York 10154

Fernando E. Viteri, M.D.
Department of Nutritional Sciences
College of Natural Resources
University of California
Berkeley, California 94720

Tomas Walter, M.D.
Institute of Nutrition and Food Technology
University of Chile
15138 Santiago 11, Chile

Philip A. Walravens, M.D.
Department of Pediatrics
University of Colorado
Health Sciences Center
Denver, Colorado 80262

Ray Yip, M.D., M.P.H.
Division of Nutrition
Center for Chronic Disease
*   Prevention and Health Promotion*
Centers for Disease Control
Atlanta, Georgia 30333

Ekhard E. Ziegler, M.D.
Department of Pediatrics
College of Medicine
University of Iowa
Iowa City, Iowa 52242

Dietary Iron: Birth to Two Years

Dietary Iron: Birth to Two Years,
edited by L. J. Filer, Jr.
Raven Press, Ltd., New York © 1989.

Review of Iron Metabolism

Peter R. Dallman

*Department of Pediatrics, University of California at San Francisco,
San Francisco, California 94143*

We understand more about iron metabolism during infancy than we did just a few years ago, and much of this progress has come from the contributions of participants at this Symposium. Iron deficiency is now recognized to affect not only hemoglobin concentration, but other essential iron proteins. Deficits in these compounds are associated with many abnormalities of body function (1,2). Iron absorption studies have clarified the critical role of the form of iron in food and the effect on iron bioavailability of food combinations, and they have been of great practical importance. These food interactions have more influence on iron nutrition than the actual amount of dietary iron (3–7). The types of diets and circumstances that lead to iron deficiency in infants have gradually been identified (8–12). Most important, this information has been rapidly applied and has had a major influence on infant feeding. As a result, there has been a drastic decline in the prevalence of iron deficiency in the past 10 to 15 years (13,14). Since the basis for this progress is a growing understanding of iron metabolism in infants (15), it is appropriate to begin with a brief review of this topic.

IRON IN THE BODY: DISTRIBUTION AND METABOLIC FUNCTION

The total amount of iron in the body of an adult is slightly less than the weight of a 5¢ coin, about 3.5 g for men (1). The major iron constituents are shown in Fig. 1 (16). These compounds are conveniently grouped into one of two categories: the first group is referred to as *essential* iron because these compounds fulfill well-defined physiological functions. The second category is referred to as *storage* iron because its major role involves the regulation of iron homeostasis and the maintenance of a reserve that assures an adequate supply of iron for production of essential iron compounds.

The term *iron deficiency* generally refers to impairment of the production of essential iron compounds due to lack of iron. When essential iron com-

1

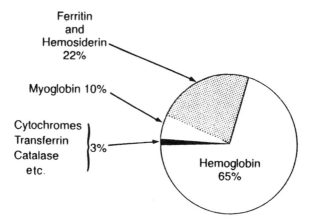

FIG. 1. Distribution of iron in humans (adult male: 3.5 g). (Reproduced from ref. 16 with permission, W.B. Saunders, © 1987.)

pounds are present in suboptimal concentrations, impaired physiological function may be anticipated even though such impairment may not be apparent. *Low iron stores per se* indicate that an individual is vulnerable to iron deficiency, but as long as the production of essential iron compounds remains intact, there are no known physiological handicaps.

The *essential iron compounds* include hemoglobin, which functions in the transport of oxygen from the lung to tissues, and mitochondrial iron proteins (the cytochromes and iron–sulfur proteins), which are essential for the oxidative production of cellular energy in the form of adenosine triphosphate (ATP).

Hemoglobin is the most familiar of the essential iron compounds. Iron first became firmly associated with blood when Menghini in the mid-1700s showed that powdered dried blood could be lifted with a magnet. Hemoglobin is now known to account for over two-thirds of the iron in the body and almost all of the iron in blood. Its concentration is easily measured in a blood sample, and this measurement is the keystone in the evaluation of iron nutrition. Age-related changes in hemoglobin concentration were first recognized in the late 19th century. Subsequently, in 1916, Williamson employed quantitative spectrophotometric methods to determine hemoglobin values in a large population that included infants (17). More precise data with confidence limits were published in the 1930s for both term and preterm infants, but these were derived mainly from lower socioeconomic groups. Recently, it has become customary to use reference values that have been obtained from representative healthy infants in whom iron deficiency and hemoglobinopathies have been excluded by laboratory studies (15).

Storage iron compounds (1) consist of ferritin and hemosiderin, which are present primarily in the liver, reticuloendothelial cells, and erythroid precursors of the bone marrow. In 1912, Ashby identified the liver as the organ that has the most to do with iron storage (18). He concluded that "when the iron is needed, it is given by the liver into the blood . . . and used to make new hemoglobin and red blood corpuscles." He also found that the concentration of liver iron was higher at birth than in the adult but that it declined rapidly during early infancy.

The total amount of storage iron can vary over a wide range without apparent impairment of body function (1). Storage iron may be almost entirely depleted before iron deficiency anemia develops. Conversely, a more than 20-fold increase in iron stores may occur before tissue damage due to iron overload becomes evident. In healthy individuals, serum ferritin reflects storage iron to a surprising degree. Thus, measurement of both serum ferritin and hemoglobin reflects the status of almost 90% of body iron.

IRON BALANCE

Almost all iron compounds in the body are continuously broken down and resynthesized (1,15). The iron that is released is very efficiently conserved and reutilized. An important consequence of this recycling is that very little iron is lost from the body on a daily basis, except when bleeding occurs. The maintenance of iron balance in adults merely requires that the amount of iron absorbed from the diet be roughly equal to what is lost from the body. The amount of iron exchanged with the environment each day is a minute percentage of total body iron. In adult men, normal iron losses in the feces, sweat, and sloughed cells amount to about 0.9 mg/day, equivalent to less than 0.1% of iron stores and an even smaller percentage of total body iron. This amount is readily absorbed from most diets. Women in their childbearing years must absorb an average of 1.3 mg/day to make up for the additional iron loss in menstrual blood. Women whose menstrual blood loss is unusually heavy and/or whose diet contains little absorbable iron are at risk of developing iron deficiency.

In infants and children, a large amount of iron is required for growth, i.e., substantially more iron must be absorbed than is lost from the body (Fig. 2) (19). For example, a 1-year-old infant loses about 0.2 mg of iron/day, calculated on the basis of body surface area from values measured in adults. The amount needed for growth averages roughly 0.6 mg. Consequently, about 75% of the 0.8 mg of absorbed iron needed per day during this period is for growth.

Regulation of Body Iron

The major factor that regulates the amount of iron in the body is intestinal absorption, which can vary over a more than 50-fold range. The bioavailability of iron—i.e., the amount absorbed from food—is determined

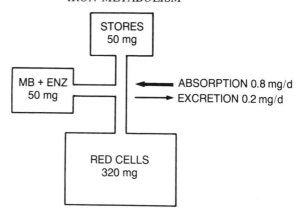

FIG. 2. Iron metabolism in the 1-year-old infant. Iron absorption must exceed iron loss to allow for growth; however, daily iron absorption and loss, even in infancy, is normally a minute percentage of total body iron. MB + ENZ = myoglobin and enzyme iron. (Reproduced from ref. 19 with permission from Hanley & Belfus, © 1988.)

both by the nature of the diet and by regulatory mechanisms in the intestinal mucosa that reflect the physiological need for iron (3,4). Iron losses can also be modulated to some extent, since intestinal losses are roughly four times higher than normal in individuals with very high iron stores.

Intestinal Regulation

The regulation of iron entry into the body takes place in the mucosal cell of the small intestine. The mechanism for this regulation is still unclear but is an area of active investigation (20–22). In infancy, the abundance of lactoferrin, the iron-binding protein in human milk, and the presence of lactoferrin receptors on the surface of the intestinal mucosa may explain why iron is so well absorbed from human milk (22). It is apparent that iron absorption is inversely related to the abundance of iron stores. If iron stores are low, as is true for most women and children, the intestinal mucosa readily takes up iron and increases the proportion absorbed from the diet. Conversely, the high iron stores typical of men and elderly women are associated with a reduced percentage of absorbed iron. These homeostatic responses protect the body to a remarkable degree from both iron deficiency and iron overload.

The homeostatic regulation of iron absorption is most effective in the physiological ranges of iron intake and iron stores. During the first postnatal months, when neonatal iron stores are typically abundant, iron absorption is depressed (23). Subsequently, iron absorption increases to accommodate the continued rapid growth that results in diminished iron stores. At all ages, the more iron that is ingested, the less the percentage but the greater the absolute amount that is absorbed.

Absorption of Iron from Foods

Quantitative estimates of iron absorption began in the 1930s and were based on classical balance studies in which the dietary intake of a nutrient was compared with fecal and urinary losses. This method was cumbersome, unpleasant, and not particularly precise with respect to iron balance. Since most food iron is unabsorbed and appears primarily in the stool, small errors in stool collection and iron analysis could lead to large discrepancies in estimation of iron retention. In addition, errors result from the loss of iron from the body into the intestinal lumen. Despite these handicaps, the early balance studies indicated that iron-rich foods did not necessarily improve iron nutrition. Spinach and egg yolk had been widely recommended as good sources of iron, but iron from both was shown to be poorly retained by infants (24). On the other hand, iron-poor human milk was associated with a more positive iron balance than cow milk. These somewhat tentative conclusions were later confirmed when more precise isotopic methods of iron absorption were developed in the 1970s (15).

There are two types of iron in food. *Heme iron,* which is present in hemoglobin and myoglobin, is supplied mainly by meat and rarely accounts for more than 10% to 15% of dietary iron. Heme iron is relatively well absorbed, and its absorption is only slightly influenced by other constituents of the diet (3,4). Most dietary iron is present in the form of *non-heme iron.* Since infant diets contain little meat, virtually all dietary iron is in the non-heme form. The absorption of non-heme iron depends on how soluble it becomes in the intestine, and this in turn is determined by the composition of foods consumed in a meal (3,4). Absorption of the small amount of iron in human milk is uniquely high, 50% on average, in contrast to about 10% of iron from unfortified cow's milk formula and 4% from iron-fortified cow's milk formula (6,7,25,26).

Studies of iron absorption from various representative meals have been carried out primarily in adults (3,4), but the results are also pertinent to the transitional diet of late infancy. For example, adults absorb about four times more non-heme iron from an entire mixed meal when the major protein source is meat, fish, or chicken, in comparison to the dairy products milk, cheese, or eggs. The beverage consumed with the meal plays an equally important role. Compared with water, orange juice will double the absorption of non-heme iron from the entire meal, whereas tea will decrease it by 75%, and milk will decrease it to a lesser degree.

The major enhancers of non-heme iron absorption are ascorbic acid and meat, fish, and poultry. Ascorbic acid is particularly important in the infant's diet (5). Some major inhibitors of absorption are bran, polyphenols (in some vegetables), and phosphate. The basis for the excellent absorption of iron from human milk is not known. The lower phosphate and protein content of human milk compared to cow's milk and the high concentration of the iron-binding protein lactoferrin (22) probably play important roles.

EFFECTS OF MATERNAL IRON DEFICIENCY ON THE FETUS AND NEWBORN

For some time, there has been scattered evidence that anemia during pregnancy was associated with a poor neonatal outcome (27–29). Recent studies provide further support for this possibility (30,31). Probably the most convincing evidence comes from a recent report by Murphy et al., who collected data on more than 54,000 pregnancies of virtually all pregnant women in the Cardiff area of Wales (30). Low birth weight, preterm delivery, and perinatal mortality were all increased when women were anemic during the first half of pregnancy. Although iron deficiency is not the only cause of anemia in pregnancy, it is by far the most common cause during the first half of gestation. Consequently, there is enough evidence that iron deficiency might carry a risk of adverse consequences during pregnancy to warrant a more focused, prospective study of iron nutrition in a large population.

Additional clues suggest that even minor impairments of oxygen transport might predispose to low birth weight in women who live at a high altitude or who smoke cigarettes. In a study of over 12 million birth records, U.S. neonates born at an altitude of > 2,500 m (primarily in Colorado) had a more than twofold higher prevalence of low birth weight compared to those born at sea level (32). Hypoxia is regarded as the most likely mechanism. Cigarette smoking results in the conversion of a small fraction of normal hemoglobin to carboxyhemoglobin, which cannot function in oxygen delivery. This abnormality may contribute to the higher prevalence of low-birth-weight infants among women who smoke (33). Although these analogies between anemia, altitude, and smoking may seem tenuous, they are in accord with the hypothesis that maintenance of optimal oxygen delivery is an important factor in the outcome of pregnancy.

Although iron deficiency is definitely associated with impaired hemoglobin production in the pregnant woman, there is little evidence that maternal iron deficiency results in significant anemia in the newborn (34–39). Even in one study that showed hemoglobin concentration to be decreased in the newborn, it was far less depressed than in the mother (40). Numerous studies, using serum ferritin as an estimate of neonatal iron stores, also showed little or no difference in offspring of mothers with mild to moderate iron deficiency compared to those who were either iron-sufficient and/or iron-supplemented. It is therefore reasonable to conclude that infants of iron-deficient mothers show little or no laboratory evidence of iron deficiency even though they might prove to have a slightly lower average birth weight. Only under the special circumstances of infants of diabetic mothers and in other situations involving placental insufficiency does the risk of neonatal iron deficiency appear to be substantial (41).

PERIODS OF GREATEST VULNERABILITY
TO IRON DEFICIENCY FOR INFANTS

Hemoglobin concentrations are normally higher at birth than at any other time of life as a result of the adaptation of the fetus to the hypoxic environment of the uterus (15,42). In addition, neonatal reserves of storage iron are relatively generous. Consequently, most newborn infants are well supplied with iron. Between birth and 4 months of age, there is almost no change in total body iron in the term infant. The need for exogenous iron is therefore modest during this period (Fig. 3). The abundant iron stores present at birth help to provide for synthesis of hemoglobin, myoglobin, and enzyme iron during the first 4 months. Additional iron from hemoglobin breakdown is also made available to meet iron needs because the concentration of hemoglobin declines from a mean of 17.0 g/dl at birth to a low of 11.0 g/dl at 2

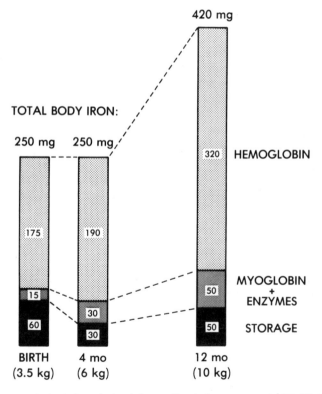

FIG. 3. Changes in body iron during infancy. Needs for exogenous iron are minimal until about 4 months of age because there is little or no increase in total body iron during this period. In contrast, large amounts of iron must be assimilated during the remainder of infancy to allow for a rapid increase in total body iron. (Reproduced from ref. 42 with permission, Almquist & Wiksell Periodical Co., © 1986.)

months of age. This low point used to be called the early anemia of infancy and was distinguished from the "late anemia of infancy" because it was unresponsive to iron treatment.

After about 4 months of age, a gradual shift occurs from an abundance of iron to the marginal iron reserves that characterize the period of continued rapid growth. This window of vulnerability to iron deficiency is the major focus of this book. The transition from feast to famine in respect to iron is primarily due to the large amount of iron required to maintain a near constant mean hemoglobin concentration of 12.5 g/dl within a rapidly expanding blood volume between 4 and 12 months. A large amount of iron, about 0.8 mg/day, must be absorbed from the diet during this period. The rate and extent to which storage iron becomes depleted can be estimated from changes in the concentration of serum ferritin and depends both on the magnitude of iron storage at birth and on the postnatal diet.

Among the first to recognize the vulnerability of infants to iron deficiency was Helen Mackay, who in 1928 reported a longitudinal study of 541 infants from a low socioeconomic group in the East End of London (43). Her influential paper showed a clear distinction between the early and late anemia of infants; only the late anemia that occurred after about 5 months of age responded to iron treatment. Late anemia was shown to be substantially milder in breast-fed infants than in infants fed a cow's milk formula. She concluded that "the excellent results of treatment with iron preparations . . . point unmistakably to iron deficiency as the factor of paramount importance in the late anemia of infancy." She also pioneered the iron fortification of cow's milk, thereby laying the foundation of our present success in preventing iron deficiency in infants.

Mackay's observations (43) still apply to term infants. Iron deficiency is apt to develop after 4 to 6 months unless there is some extra source of iron in the diet in addition to human milk or unfortified formula (15). Low-birth-weight infants start out with a lower absolute amount of storage iron than term infants, since neonatal iron stores are roughly proportional to body weight (10). In addition, their postnatal iron needs are greater to allow for a more rapid rate of growth. Consequently, low-birth-weight infants deplete their iron stores by 2 to 3 months unless they receive an iron supplement if they are fed human milk or unless they receive an iron-fortified formula (10). If frequent blood samples are taken for laboratory studies, iron stores are likely to become depleted earlier.

LOOKING TO THE FUTURE

Up to this point, our discussion has dealt with what we have already learned about factors that are important in maintaining iron homeostasis during infancy. Little has been mentioned about the mechanisms by which the intestinal mucosa regulates iron absorption and by which tissue cells adjust their iron uptake. Although regulation of iron absorption by the intestine is still not well understood (20–22), a great deal of progress is being made in understanding how cells take up an appropriate amount of iron from serum transferrin (18,44,45). Transferrin, the serum iron-binding protein, plays an essential role in transporting iron between sites of absorption, storage, and utilization (44,45). Cell surface membranes contain a specific transferrin receptor that serves as the chief means of iron uptake. These receptors are most abundant in tissues, such as red cell precursors, liver, and placenta, which have a high need for iron. The number of receptors is highly regulated. When cells are in an iron-rich environment, the number of receptors is decreased (44,45). Conversely, in iron-poor surroundings, the number of transferrin receptors is increased. These changes in receptor number can be accounted for by corresponding alterations in the level of messenger RNA. Such alterations in turn are mediated by two regions of the gene that can produce more than 20-fold differences in transcription levels depending on iron availability. Interestingly, this exciting area of research is focused more on the question of how environmental changes affect gene expression than on iron metabolism. However, studies in this area may also bring about radical changes in our future perception of iron metabolism and iron nutrition.

REFERENCES

1. Bothwell, T. H., Charlton, R. W., Cook, J. D., and Finch, C. A. (1979): *Iron Metabolism in Man.* Blackwell Scientific Publications, Oxford.
2. Dallman, P. R. (1986): Biochemical basis for manifestations of iron deficiency. *Annu. Rev. Nutr.,* 6:13–40.
3. Hallberg, L. (1981): Bioavailability of dietary iron in man. *Annu. Rev. Nutr.,* 1:123–147.
4. Charlton, R. W., and Bothwell, T. H. (1983): Iron absorption. *Annu. Rev. Med.* 34:55–68.
5. Cook, J. D., and Bothwell, T. H. (1984): Availability of iron from infant food. In: *Nutrition in Infancy and Childhood,* edited by A. Stekel. Raven Press, New York, pp. 119–143.
6. Saarinen, U. M., Siimes, M. A., and Dallman, P. R. (1977): Iron absorption in infants. High bioavailability of breast milk iron as indicated by the extrinsic tag method of iron absorption and by the concentration of serum ferritin. *J. Pediatr.,* 91:36–39.
7. McMillan, J. A., Landaw, S. A., and Oski, F. A. (1976): Iron sufficiency in breast-fed infants and the availability of iron from human milk. *Pediatrics,* 58:686–691.
8. Saarinen, U. M. (1978): Need for iron supplementation in infants on prolonged breast feeding. *J. Pediatr.,* 93:177–180.
9. Oski, F. A., and Landaw, S. A. (1980): Inhibition of iron absorption from human milk by baby food. *Am. J. Dis. Child.,* 134:459–460.
10. Lundström, U., Siimes, M. A., and Dallman, P. R. (1977): At what age does iron supplementation become necessary in low-birth-weight infants? *J. Pediatr.,* 91:878–883.
11. Fomon, S. J., Ziegler, E. E., Nelson, S. E., and Edwards, B. B. (1981): Cow's milk feeding in infancy: gastrointestinal blood loss and iron nutritional status. *J. Pediatr.,* 98:540–545.
12. Sadowitz, P. D., and Oski, F. A. (1983): Iron status and infant feeding practices in an urban ambulatory center. *Pediatrics,* 72:33–36.
13. Yip, R., Binkin, N. J., Fleshood, L., and Trowbridge, F. L. (1987): Declining prevalence of anemia among low-income children in the United States. *J.A.M.A.,* 258:1619–1623.
14. Yip, R., Walsh, K. M., Goldfarb, M. G., and Binkin, N. J. (1987): Declining prevalence of anemia in childhood. A pediatric success story? *Pediatrics,* 80:330–334.

15. Dallman, P. R., Siimes, M. A., and Stekel, A. (1980): Iron deficiency in infancy and childhood. *Am. J. Clin. Nutr.*, 33:86–118.
16. Dallman, P. R. (1987): Iron deficiency and related nutritional anemias. In: *Hematology of Infancy and Childhood*, 3rd ed., edited by D. G. Nathan and F. A. Oski. W. B. Saunders, Philadelphia, 276.
17. Williamson, C. S. (1916): Influence of age and sex on hemoglobin. A spectrophotometric analysis of 919 cases. *Arch. Intern. Med.*, 18:505–528.
18. Ashby, H. T. (1912): The relation of iron to anemia in infancy and childhood. *Lancet*, 2:150–153.
19. Dallman, P. R. (1988): Nutritional anemia of infancy: iron, folic acid, and B12. In: *Nutrition During Infancy*, edited by R. Tsang and B. Nichols. Hanley & Belfus, Philadelphia, 219.
20. Huebers, H. A., and Finch, C. A. (1987): The physiology of transferrin and transferrin receptors. *Physiol. Rev.*, 67:520–581.
21. Peters, T. J., Raja, K. B., Simpson, R. J., and Snape, S. (1988): Mechanisms and regulation of iron absorption. *Ann. N.Y. Acad. Sci.*, 526:141–147.
22. Davidson, L. A., and Lonnerdal, B. (1988): Specific binding of lactoferrin to brush-border membrane: ontogeny and effect of glycon chain. *Am. J. Physiol.*, 254:G580–G585.
23. Götze, C., Schafer, K. H., Heinrich, H. C., and Bartels, H. (1970): Eisenstoffwechselstudien an fruhgeborenen und gesunden reifgeborenen wahrend des ersten lebensjahres it dem ganzkorperzahler und anderen methoden. *Monatschr Kinderheilk* 118:210.
24. Stearns, G., and Stringer, D. (1937): Iron retention in infancy. *J. Nutr.*, 13:127–141.
25. Rios, E., Hunter, R. E., Cook, J. D., et al. (1975): The absorption of iron as supplements in infant cereal and infant formulas. *Pediatrics*, 55:686–693.
26. Saarinen, U. M., and Siimes, M. A. (1977): Iron absorption from infant formula and the optimal level of iron supplementation. *Acta Paediatr. Scand.*, 66:719–722.
27. Klein, L. (1962): Premature birth and maternal prenatal anemia. *Am. J. Obstet. Gynecol.*, 83:588–590.
28. Macgregor, M. W. (1963): Maternal anaemia as a factor in prematurity and perinatal mortality. *Scot. Med. J.*, 8:134–140.
29. Nhonoli, A. M., Kihama, F. E., and Famji, B. D. (1975): The relation between maternal and cord serum iron levels and its effect on fetal growth in iron deficient mothers without malarial infection. *Br. J. Obstet. Gynaecol.*, 82:467–470.
30. Murphy, J. F., O'Riordan, J., Newcombe, R. G., Coles, E. C., and Pearson, J. F. (1986): Relation of haemoglobin levels in first and second trimesters to outcome of pregnancy. *Lancet*, 1:992–995.
31. Lieberman, E., Ryan, K. J., Monson, R. R., and Schoenbaum, S. C. (1987): Risk factors accounting for racial differences in the rate of premature birth. *N. Engl. J. Med.*, 317:743–748.
32. Yip, R. (1987): Altitude and birth weight. *J. Pediatr.*, 111:869–876.
33. Pirani, B. B. K., and MacGillivray, I. (1978): Smoking during pregnancy. Its effects on maternal metabolism and fetomaternal function. *Obstet. Gynecol.*, 52:257–263.
34. Sisson, T. R. C., and Lund, C. J. (1958): The influence of maternal iron deficiency on the newborn. *Am. J. Clin. Nutr.*, 6:376–384.
35. Sturgeon, P. (1959): Studies of iron requirements in infants. III. Influence of supplemental iron during normal pregnancy on mother and infant. B. The infant. *Br. J. Haematol.*, 5:45–55.
36. DeLeeuw, N. K. M., Lowenstein, L., and Hsieh, Y. S. (1966): Iron deficiency and hydremia in normal pregnancy. *Medicine*, 45:291–315.
37. Murray, M. J., Murray, A. B., Murray, N. J., and Murray, M. B. (1978): The effect of iron status of Nigerian mothers on that of their infants at birth and six months and on the concentration of iron in breast milk. *Br. J. Nutr.*, 39:627–630.
38. Agrawal, R. M. D., Tripathi, A. M., and Agarwal, K. N. (1983): Cord blood haemoglobin, iron and ferritin status in maternal anaemia. *Acta Paediatr. Scand.*, 72:545–548.
39. Dawson, E. B., and McGanity, W. J. (1987): Protection of maternal iron stores in pregnancy. *J. Reprod. Med.*, 32(suppl):475–496.
40. Singla, P. N., Schand, S., Khanna, S., and Agarwal, K. N. (1978): Effect of maternal anaemia on the placenta and the newborn infant. *Acta Paediatr. Scand.*, 67:645–648.
41. Chockalingam, U. M., Murphy, E., Ophoven, J. C., Weisdorf, S. A., and Georgieff, M. K. (1987): Cord transferrin and ferritin values in newborn infants at risk for prenatal uteroplacental insufficiency and chronic hypoxia. *J. Pediatr.*, 111:283–286.
42. Dallman, P. R. (1986): Iron deficiency in the weanling: a nutritional problem on the way to resolution. *Acta Paediatr. Scand.*, 323:59–67.

43. Mackay, H. M. (1928): Anaemia in infancy; prevalence and prevention. *Arch. Dis. Child.,* 3:117–146.
44. Casey, J. L., Hentze, M. W., Koeller, D. M., et al. (1988): Iron-responsive elements: regulatory RNA sequences that control mRNA levels and translation. *Science,* 240:924–928.
45. Casey, J. L., DiJeso, B., Rao, K., Rouault, T. A., Klausner, R. D., and Harford, J. B. (1988): The promoter region of the human transferrin receptor gene. *Ann. N.Y. Acad. Sci.,* 526:54–64.

Dietary Iron: Birth to Two Years,
edited by L. J. Filer, Jr.
Raven Press, Ltd., New York © 1989.

Discussion

Dr. Filer: In Dr. Bothwell's study on the influence of iron stores on iron absorption, were these absorptions measured with a test dose?

Dr. Dallman: The dose consisted of 3 mg of ferrous iron after an overnight fast. The fasting conditions and the relatively low dose help to explain why the absorption values are very high. The subjects were also fasted for 4 hr after the dose was given, so it was not a way to determine actual iron absorption under normal dietary circumstances. Nevertheless, this study does establish that there is a very strict relationship between the ability of the intestinal mucosa to absorb iron and body iron stores.

Dr. Owen: How much of the iron in bone marrow is non-heme?

Dr. Dallman: Much of the iron in the marrow is in developing red blood cells and is not stainable. This includes non-heme iron in the form of ferritin, but also heme iron in the form of newly synthesized hemoglobin. The stainable iron is primarily in reticuloendothelial cells, and consists mostly of ferritin and hemosiderin (non-heme iron). The liver contains much more iron than the bone marrow. In most circumstances, with the exception of hemochromatosis and certain other diseases, bone marrow non-heme iron reflects the much larger liver iron stores.

Dr. Oski: What is the evidence for regulation of iron absorption during the first few months of life when infants have very high serum ferritin levels and are absorbing iron?

Dr. Dallman: Heinrich and co-workers have measured iron absorption in premature and full-term infants at various ages. They showed very clearly that iron absorption was lower in the 1-month-old infant than in the infant at 2 and 3 months of age. This indicates that the regulatory factors that characterize adults must also apply in the infant. At 1 or 2 months of age, when there are high transferrin saturations and fairly high iron stores like those in the adult male, iron absorption is as low as in the adult male. It is only later in infancy, when iron stores become depleted and there is a need for iron, that absorption increases.

Dr. Ziegler: Do you interpret the data on iron absorption in infants as indicating that as the infant gets older, his iron nutritional status declines and that this triggers iron absorption? Do we actually know that this is the mechanism?

Dr. Dallman: The simplest explanation is that iron stores affect iron absorption; however, it could also involve some other phenomenon such as gut maturation.

A study from Israel, where tea is commonly given to young children, has indicated that tea inhibits iron absorption. Do young children in China commonly drink tea?

Dr. Yip: It is quite common in Moslem cultures.

Dr. Dallman: Since the Infant Formula Act was passed, formula that is called "unfortified" still has some added iron in it. How much iron does the Infant Formula Act require for low-iron formula?

Dr. Filer: The Infant Formula Act now requires a minimum of 0.15 mg of iron/100 kcal, but enough may be added to provide about 1.4 or 1.6 mg/liter.

Dr. Owen: The amount of iron declared on the label is 1.5 mg/liter and, according to our analytical data, this is an accurate value. I think that 1.5 mg is added to that naturally present in formula, which is probably around 0.2 or 0.3 mg. Iron levels rarely exceed 1.6 or 1.7 mg/liter.

Dr. Dallman: In the U.S., it is common to add 12 mg/liter of iron-fortified formula. Based on a study that was done by Siimes and co-workers, many European countries add about 6 mg of iron/liter. This study indicated that as more iron is added to the formula, the percentage of iron that is absorbed decreases. Consequently, almost as much iron is absorbed from a formula containing 6 mg of iron/liter as from one with 12 mg/liter. It may be time to reexamine the merits of the 6-mg level again, because there are increasing concerns about not using more iron than is necessary to prevent iron deficiency.

Dr. Oski: What is the difference between 6 and 12 mg of added iron in terms of its effect on zinc bioavailability?

Dr. Dallman: We do not know.

Dr. Walter: We studied formulas containing 1.5 or 1.6 mg of iron versus 15 mg of iron. There were no differences in serum zinc concentrations.

Dr. Ziegler: We have carried out metabolic balance studies with 3 versus 10.5 mg of iron and found no difference in zinc balance.

Dr. Walravens: There is enough zinc added to formulas so that as long as one remains within a reasonable Fe/Zn ratio (3:1), the iron levels in current use are safe. The problem with zinc lies in the measurement of zinc status. Unless blood is drawn after fasting, we do not know how to interpret plasma zinc values. If a formula contains 5 mg of zinc and 6 or 12 mg of iron, it is probably all right.

Dr. Dallman: I suspect that zinc–iron interactions are going to be demonstrable when we have more sensitive ways to measure them. We know that they occur in animals and we know that they occur under extreme situations. Bo Lonnerdal has recently emphasized the value of looking at ratios of nutrients, especially iron, copper, and zinc.

Dr. Filer: As a general rule, such ratios must be distorted considerably before there is an effect.

Dr. Dallman: If one uses human milk as a frame of reference, the ratios are going to be distorted somewhat. To some extent, one can justify that because iron is not as well absorbed from cow's milk as it is from human milk. We may need about four times as much iron in cow's milk-based formulas to get an equivalent amount of absorbed iron. Even so, whether one considers how much is in the diet or how much is absorbed, the concept of ratios is an effective one that we will hear more and more about.

Dr. Filer: Dr. Walravens, would you have more concern about the copper–zinc ratio than the iron–zinc ratio?

Dr. Walravens: Probably yes. There have been more demonstrated cases of borderline copper deficiency with high-dose zinc supplements that have been taken to increase statural growth. In studies of sickle-cell patients given 100 to 150 mg of zinc/day, there was a dramatic decrease in ceruloplasmin levels. If there is 0.6 mg of copper and 5 mg of zinc/liter of formula, this is a ninefold ratio. There shouldn't be too much concern about that ratio. A 100-fold ratio would certainly be damaging. Dr. Ziegler, have you had experience with copper in balance studies?

Dr. Ziegler: Yes. In the study that I mentioned earlier, we observed lower copper absorption with higher iron intakes but we also had the problem of having two different levels of zinc that had no effect on copper. The Zn/Cu ratios were much lower than 30 to 1.

Dr. Dallman: Regarding this issue of whether we can do with less iron in formulas, it is easy to consider it a matter of, "If it ain't broke, don't fix it." We have been so pleased with the fact that the present level of iron prevents iron deficiency that there has been little pressure to see if less will work. However, many European companies are now using less iron. In addition, there is concern about excess iron being a predisposing factor to infection and to undesirable nutrient interaction. For these reasons, we need to find out whether smaller amounts of iron in infant formulas are just as effective in preventing iron deficiency.

Dr. Walter: The only concern that I have about a specific recommendation for decreasing the iron in formula is that in some countries there is no other source of iron other than formula. In our studies, iron deficiency and low iron stores occur even with 15 mg of iron per liter because there is no other source of iron in the diet.

Dr. Dallman: Of course, you used a full-fat powdered milk that is higher in calcium and phosphorus than the formulas used in the U.S. What applies to the U.S. and Europe may need to be modified in other settings and according to the composition of the formula.

Dr. Filer: Full-fat powdered milk is also higher in protein.

Dr. Dallman: So there is a potential for inhibition that might not exist when using formulas.

Dr. Filer: Lowering the level of iron contained in infant formulas may be a concern in very low-income families who overdilute the formula or don't feed the formula at regular strength and therefore the infant gets less iron. Such examples might be found in developing countries. Pediatricians in

Spanish Harlem in New York City might have concerns about lowering of the iron level of formula products.

Dr. Dallman: I am not sure that it would justify industry-wide levels of fortification to accommodate that tiny portion of the population.

Dr. Filer: We have almost 20 years of experience with the 12 mg addition of iron, but I do not believe we have any evidence of either imbalance with any other metal or problems with iron toxicity even in subtle forms.

Dr. Dallman: I agree, but I think it is more an issue of where the "burden of proof" lies.

Dr. Filer: As an investigator, I welcome your recommendation that it be studied. However, I then ask myself the following questions: Where does one study such a problem? Does one go to Chile or China to study the effectiveness of this lowered level of iron fortification? Or does one go to Canada, where, from what I understand, very little iron-containing formula is used at all? There are lots of places to study such a proposal, so I don't think that is a problem. I wonder what thoughts Frank Oski has about this issue.

Dr. Oski: Personally, I think that if 6 mg of iron is effective (and based on balance studies it is), there is no reason to add 12 mg.

Dr. Dallman: The next step is to verify the balance studies by doing actual field or clinical trials to establish the efficacy of the lower dose. I am not aware of any carefully done European studies that actually show that a 6-mg dose is effective.

Dr. Owen: If such are published, they are in obscure journals, since I am not able to find such published reports.

Dr. Ziegler: Didn't Hashke and co-workers publish a paper on this topic?

Dr. Owen: They studied levels of 6 or 8 mg of iron per liter of formula. However, these studies were complicated by feeding meat and beikost. I don't recall any studies that used formula as the sole source of nutrition.

Dr. Ziegler: In the study of pregnant women in Southern Wales, how do you explain the results showing that higher hemoglobin concentrations are associated with poorer pregnancy outcomes?

Dr. Dallman: The higher hemoglobin concentrations were thought to result from failure of the plasma volume to expand normally. This hormonally regulated phenomenon is very important for a healthy pregnancy. Women who have a high hemoglobin concentration are at increased risk of hypertension and pre-eclampsia. The elevation in hemoglobin levels is unrelated to iron metabolism.

Dr. Yip: The risk factors or problems associated with poor pregnancy outcomes are often associated with nutritional problems and anemia. With this type of information, it is hard to tell whether anemia or high hemoglobin levels are contributory or causative factors for the poor pregnancy outcomes or whether these outcomes are the result of poor general health. The data are suggestive that there is a strong association between pregnancy outcome and these hematological changes; however, the exact relationship is difficult to determine.

Dr. Dallman: I think it has to be emphasized that when relationships like these are observed, the next question is whether or not it is due to iron. It is true that iron deficiency is the most common cause of anemia in early pregnancy. Later in pregnancy, one must also consider urinary tract infection and other possibilities. The task, now, is to do a large prospective study in pregnant women to compare a group of women receiving iron supplementation with a group of women who are not and to determine the outcome of the pregnancy.

Dr. Filer: Could you comment on the old "mucosal block" theory? If the regulation of iron uptake takes place at the genome level of the cell, as you indicated, we would still have the "mucosal block" situation.

Dr. Dallman: I don't think that there ever was anything wrong with the "mucosal block" idea. It was a description of what happens rather than an explanation of how it happens, and the description is still largely correct. If the individual has large liver iron stores and a lot of iron in the intestinal mucosa, not very much iron is going to be absorbed, and one can call that a "block." If the reverse is true, as in iron depletion, the individual absorbs a lot of iron. So, in a sense, the term "block" is still an attractive term. It exaggerates the effect and does not explain its cause. But it is an effective description of what happens.

Dr. Ziegler: Is the absorption of heme iron influenced by the iron status of the individual?

Dr. Dallman: It probably is to some extent, but much less than the absorption of non-heme iron. I believe that the range over which heme iron can be absorbed may be about fourfold, whereas the range of non-heme iron absorption is more than 50-fold. Therefore, there is a much broader regulatory range with non-heme iron.

Dietary Iron: Birth to Two Years,
edited by L. J. Filer, Jr.
Raven Press, Ltd., New York © 1989.

Iron Nutritional Status Defined

Ray Yip

*Division of Nutrition, Center for Chronic Disease Prevention and Health Promotion,
Centers for Disease Control, Atlanta, Georgia 30333*

In general, the determination of iron deficiency is based on laboratory testing. Obvious clinical signs are helpful only in the diagnosis of severe iron deficiency that results in severe anemia. These signs include pallor, tachycardia, and evidence of high cardiac output. The laboratory diagnosis can be classified into two types: biochemical and hematological.

However, it is not always easy to define iron deficiency by means of laboratory tests. Iron deficiency represents a spectrum ranging from a mild form of reduced iron stores with no physiological impairment to a severe form with marked impairment of multiple organ systems including anemia. For this reason, not only is it difficult to make a clear-cut clinical diagnosis, but it has also resulted in various definitions of iron deficiency. In addition, iron biochemical tests lack a functional "gold standard" for evaluating their results properly. Although a number of tests are available for the testing of iron nutritional status, there is the lack of a single, perfect test for the diagnosis of iron deficiency. Consequently, detecting iron deficiency in a clinical or field setting is more complex than commonly perceived.

Biochemical testing for iron deficiency is based on the correlation of the deficient state, as defined by the lack of stainable bone marrow iron and a specific range of iron biochemical values. The commonly used indices include low serum iron (Fe), elevated total iron binding capacity (TIBC), low transferrin saturation (Fe/TIBC), low serum ferritin, and elevated erythrocyte protoporphyrin (EP) (Table 1). A diagnosis of iron deficiency is often based on abnormal results in one or more of these tests. Hematological tests detect hypochromic microcytic anemia among those individuals with relatively severe iron deficiency. The major hematological tests for iron deficiency and cutoff values based on the Second National Health and Nutrition Examination Survey (NHANES II) or recommended by the American Academy of Pediatrics (AAP) are listed in Table 1 (1,2).

Based on the presence or absence of anemia, a case of iron deficiency can be classified as iron deficiency anemia or iron deficiency without anemia, the latter representing the mild end of the spectrum. The concept that not all

TABLE 1. *Common laboratory tests and cutoff values*
for diagnosis of iron deficiency in young children

	Age (years)	Cutoff values	
Biochemical tests			
Serum iron (Fe)	1–2	<30 µg/dl	
	3–5	<30 µg/dl	
Total iron binding	1–2	>480 µg/dl	
capacity (TIBC)	3–5	>470 µg/dl	
Transferrin saturation	1–2	<8%	
	3–5	<9%	
Erythrocyte protoporphyrin	1–5	≥35 µg/dl whole blood	
		or ≥90 µg/dl RBC	
		or ≥3.0 µg/g of Hgb	
		or ≥90 µmol/mol of heme	
Serum ferritin	1–5	<8 to <12	
Hematologic tests		NHANES II (1)[a]	AAP (2)[b]
Hemoglobin (Hgb)	1–2	<10.7 g/dl	<11.0 g/dl
	3–5	<10.9 g/dl	<11.0 g/dl
Hematocrit (Hct)	1–2	<32%	<33%
	3–5	<32%	<34%
Mean corpuscular volume	1–2	<67 fl	<70 fl
(MCV)	3–5	<73 fl	<73 fl
Mean corpuscular Hgb	1–2	<22 pg	
(MCH)	3–5	<25 pg	
Mean corpuscular Hgb	1–2	<32 µg/dl	
concentration (MCHC)	3–5	<32 µg/dl	

[a]Reference values of −2 standard deviations from NHANES II (1).
[b]Recommended values from the American Academy of Pediatrics (2).

iron-deficient persons have anemia is important. Of equal importance is the fact that not all anemia results from iron deficiency. Anemia has many known causes; common ones include infection, inflammation, and mild hereditary anemia, such as thalassemia traits (3).

In clinical practice, hemoglobin or hematocrit is one of the most widely used tests for detecting anemia. Because of the strong association between anemia and iron deficiency, these terms are often used interchangeably. If a population has a high prevalence of iron deficiency, many individuals will have iron deficiency anemia, representing the more severe end of the spectrum (Fig. 1). Of those who are anemic in a population with a high prevalence of iron deficiency, the majority will have evidence of iron deficiency. In such a population, the loose use of "anemia" to denote iron deficiency anemia can be justified. However, in another population where iron deficiency is relatively rare, the relationship between anemia and iron deficiency may not justify the interchangeable use of these terms (Fig. 2). In a population in whom the prevalence of iron deficiency is low, most iron-deficient cases are likely to be mild and may not manifest as anemia. However, other causes of anemia, especially those that do not involve nutritional factors,

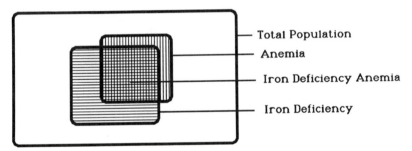

FIG. 1. Diagrammatic representation of a population with high prevalence of iron deficiency. When the prevalence of anemia is high, most cases of anemia are related to iron deficiency.

may represent the majority of the anemic cases. Therefore, in such a population, only a minority of the anemic subjects will have evidence of iron deficiency, and a distinction between anemia, iron deficiency anemia, and iron deficiency is important. Currently, in the U.S., the prevalence of childhood iron deficiency is approaching a state similar to that represented in Fig. 2. For this reason, we need to reassess the way we define, screen, and diagnose childhood iron deficiency.

LIMITATIONS OF LABORATORY TESTS FOR DETECTING IRON DEFICIENCY

A number of laboratory tests are available for determining iron deficiency, and the choice of which one to use depends largely on the purpose of the case finding as well as on the practicality of the testing circumstances. In general, a clinical screening for those individuals who have a high likelihood of iron deficiency requires a single, simple test suitable for field or outpatient settings, such as the hemoglobin or hematocrit tests. In a hospital setting, the differential diagnosis of the anemic patient often relies on iron

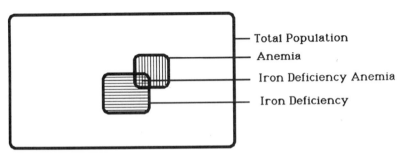

FIG. 2. Diagrammatic representation of a population with a low prevalence of iron deficiency. Only a minority of anemic subjects have evidence of iron deficiency.

biochemical tests, such as transferrin saturation or serum ferritin. However, each of the various screening and diagnostic tests has limitations. In population-based surveys, the prevalence of anemia can be determined by multiple, iron-related laboratory tests to bypass the limitations of each individual test.

Lack of Test Specificity

Although iron deficiency causes physiological alterations, including those related to the hematological system, few of these alterations produce clinical signs or pathological evidence unique to iron deficiency or detectable among milder cases. Fortunately, a few biochemical or physiological markers are relatively specific to iron nutritional status. For example, stainable bone marrow iron corresponds to body iron stores, and the increased intestinal iron absorption rate corresponds to functional iron deficiency. However, tests such as stainable bone marrow iron or iron isotope absorption are not practical clinical tools for routine evaluation. The iron biochemical tests listed in Table 1 have good correlation with iron status. However, because each of these tests can be altered by conditions other than nutritional iron status, their usefulness is somewhat limited. The most notable such condition is the inflammatory process, which causes significant disturbance of iron metabolism. As a result, alterations occur in iron biochemical tests that mimic iron deficiency, i.e., reduced serum iron, reduced transferrin saturation, and elevated EP (4,5).

Normal Test Variations

The usefulness of some iron biochemical tests is also limited because they vary significantly with normal conditions. For example, serum iron and transferrin saturation are subject to diurnal variation and to the influence of recent iron intake.

Lack of Intertest Correlations

In addition, these tests do not correlate well with each other except in the case of severe iron deficiency. Often, one test indicates iron deficiency, whereas another test may not (Fig. 3). Among the common laboratory tests for iron deficiency, there appears to be no perfect test. Part of the reason for the lack of strong correlation is that each test measures a different aspect of iron metabolism. For example, serum ferritin is an index of body iron stores, while elevated EP indicates an inadequate iron supply for heme synthesis. Because a low iron store may or may not affect iron supply for heme

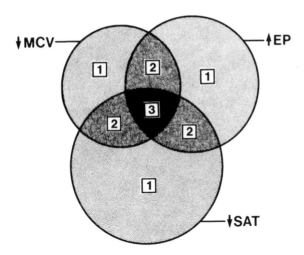

FIG. 3. Diagrammatic representation of the interaction between iron biochemical tests. Positive results from each test intersect only partially with results from other tests. The number in each segment indicates the number of positive tests. Test criteria: MCV < 73 fl; transferrin saturation < 12%; EP > 80 µg/dl of RBC. Based on data for children 1–5 years of age from the NHANES II, 1976–1980.

synthesis, a low serum ferritin result may not always be associated with an elevated EP on an individual basis.

Together, the lack of test specificity, subject to normal physiological influences, and the lack of high intertest correlation make the interpretation of laboratory test results for iron deficiency a complicated task.

THE MULTIPLE TEST APPROACH TO DEFINING IRON DEFICIENCY

Because of the limitations of each laboratory test for iron deficiency, the multiple test approach can be used in circumstances in which vigorous definition of the condition is needed (6). The basic principle of multiple testing is that for those persons with multiple abnormal test results, the certainty is high that they have iron deficiency (i.e., high positive predictive value). Conversely, for those persons with multiple normal test results, the certainty that they do not have iron deficiency is also high (high test specificity). Individuals who have three positive tests (Fig. 3) would be regarded as the most definite cases. However, because those who have all positive results represent only a small fraction of all individuals with one or more positive tests, this is a definite but restrictive definition of iron deficiency. Very restricted criteria would mean that many persons with less severe iron deficiency would be regarded as normal (i.e., low test sensitivity or a high false-negative rate), whereas broad criteria would indicate that those who have one or more positive tests would be considered to have iron deficiency. However, the broad definition would include as many non-iron deficiency cases as iron deficiency cases, although most of the true cases would also be included (high test sensitivity and a high false-positive rate).

The main advantage of multiple tests is the flexibility in choosing suitable criteria for defining iron deficiency based on multiple combinations of test results. In recent years, the iron nutritional status of the U.S. population has been characterized by the multiple test approach, using data collected by the NHANES II (7,8). The combination of three tests is often referred to as the "ferritin model": the serum ferritin, transferrin saturation, and EP tests are used together, and iron deficiency is defined as having two or more positive test results. Another approach that combines mean corpuscular volume (MCV), transferrin saturation, and EP tests is referred as the "MCV model." The main drawback of the multiple testing approach in determining iron deficiency is the high cost. Consequently, this approach is impractical for routine screening.

DEFINING THE NORMAL RANGE OF HEMATOLOGICAL AND IRON BIOCHEMICAL TESTS WITH MULTIPLE TESTING

Reference Versus Standard Criteria for Defining Cutoff Values

In general, the normal range of given laboratory values is based on the test results of the central 95% distribution of "healthy" individuals. Most clinical chemistry tests are based on this principle (9). The sample of healthy individuals, after those considered "unhealthy" are excluded, is regarded as a test standard. If a population sample is used to determine the central 95% range of a test distribution, without excluding those who are "unhealthy" or those who have abnormalities, such a sample is considered a test reference. Some nutritional criteria such as growth curves are based on a reference population. It is desirable that the sample for either a test reference or a test standard properly represents the population. The main difference between the two is that a standard represents only healthy individuals in a population. It excludes individuals with abnormal conditions, since their presence would probably result in a skewed normal range of test results.

In the development of the normal hemoglobin range or cutoff point to define anemia, individuals with a high likelihood of iron deficiency should be excluded. This is particularly important if the reference population has a high prevalence of iron deficiency, and hence a high prevalence of anemia, since this would result in a "normal" range based on a reference sample skewed to a lower hemoglobin value. A hemoglobin cutoff value from a reference sample representing a high prevalence of iron deficiency would be of little value in the screening or diagnosis of iron deficiency, because many truly anemic cases would still be above the cutoff value. Figure 4 illustrates different cutoff values based on an unselected reference versus a healthy standard sample.

Development of Normal Hematological and Iron Biochemical Test Ranges Using a Standard Sample of the U.S. Population

The second National Health and Nutrition Examination Survey, 1976–1980 (NHANES II) (7,8) is the latest and the most comprehensive nutritional characterization of the U.S. population. Over 19,000 individuals had complete hematological testing and over 17,000 individuals had iron biochemical testing, including transferrin saturation and EP. A smaller sample was also tested for serum ferritin. The NHANES II sample consisted of individuals aged 6 months to 75 years representing noninstitutional U.S. residents during the survey period (10). Because iron deficiency is the most common nutritional deficiency in the U.S. and a known contributing factor to anemia, the availability of multiple test results from the NHANES II sample allows us to develop normal test ranges based on a test standard, i.e., a population that excludes those with a high likelihood of iron deficiency.

For the development of each age- and sex-specific normal range for hematological or iron biochemical values, the exclusion of abnormal cases was based on three other tests (1), as described in Table 2. The normal range for hematological and iron biochemical tests for younger children was based on the test standard detailed in Table 3. Although the NHANES II sample did not have an adequate sample for infants younger than 12 months, the laboratory values of the 1- to 2-year age group can probably be used for infants 6 to 12 months of age.

Age-specific laboratory criteria are needed to define anemia or iron defi-

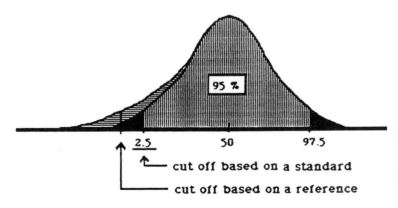

FIG. 4. Diagrammatic representation of different cutoff values based on an unselected reference sample vs. a healthy standard sample.

TABLE 2. *Exclusion criteria for test standards of laboratory tests[a]*

Laboratory tests	Exclusion criteria
Hemoglobin Hematocrit Red blood cells	MCV < 80 fl, Fe/TIBC < 16%, EP > 75 µg/dl of RBC
Mean cell volume Mean cell hemoglobin Mean corpuscular Hgb conc.	Anemia,[b] Fe/TIBC < 16%, EP > 75 µg/dl of RBC
Serum iron Total iron binding capacity Transferrin saturation	Anemia,[b] MCV < 80 fl, EP > 75 µg/dl of RBC
Erythrocyte protoporphyrin	Anemia,[b] Fe/TIBC < 16%, blood lead > 30 µg/dl

[a]Data from ref. 1.
[b]Lower limit of 95% range for hemoglobin by age and sex.

TABLE 3. *Normal range of hematological and iron biochemical tests for children 1 to 5 years of age[a]*

Test	Age (years)	Lower limit of 95% range	Median	Upper limit of 95% range
Hgb (g/dl)	1–2 3–5	10.7 10.9	12.3 12.5	13.8 14.4
Hct (%)	1–2 3–5	32 32	35.9 36.3	40 42
MCV (fl)	1–2 3–5	67 73	79 81	88 91
Fe (µg/dl)	1–2 3–5	31 28	83 88	200 163
TIBC (µg/dl)	1–2 3–5	301 299	394 377	479 472
Fe/TIBC (%)	1–2 3–5	8 9	20 23	43 45
EP (µg/dl of RBC)	1–2 3–5	36 33	59 54	100 96

[a]Based on NHANES II standard.

ciency because of the marked developmental change in these values with age among healthy children (1,2). Developmental changes of hemoglobin occur from infancy to adulthood, and hemoglobin markedly increases throughout childhood (Fig. 5). Consequently, hemoglobin cutoff values for anemia must be appropriate to age.

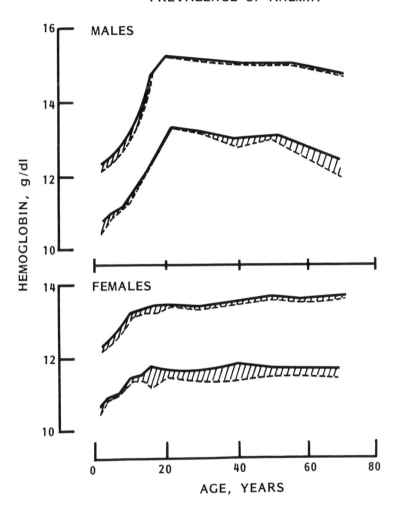

PREVALENCE OF ANEMIA

FIG. 5. Age-related changes in hemoglobin concentration. The upper lines for males and females represent the 50th percentile and the lower lines the 2.5 percentile. The solid line represents hemoglobin values after individuals with abnormal iron biochemical test results are excluded. The dotted line represents hemoglobin values before such exclusion. The shift of median hemoglobin values can be used to estimate the prevalence of anemia. Based on data from the NHANES II, 1976–1980. (Reproduced from ref. 7 with permission by the *American Journal of Clinical Nutrition*, © 1984.)

ISSUES RELATED TO RACE-SPECIFIC CRITERIA TO DEFINE ANEMIA

Findings from several large-scale U.S. nutritional surveys consistently found that blacks had lower mean hemoglobin and lower mean hematocrit values than whites at all ages (11–13). The reported differences in mean hemoglobin ranged from 0.5 to 1.5 g/dl and up to 3% of hematocrit. As a result, some investigators suggested that separate cutoff criteria be used to define anemia among blacks (13,14). The use of race-specific criteria would be appropriate if the truly "healthy" black population had a lower mean hemoglobin and if the lower hemoglobin were related to a generalized down-shift of hemoglobin distribution, i.e., all blacks require a lower hemoglobin concentration than do whites in a healthy state. However, the evidence so far does not support this thesis. Existing evidence suggests that the lower hemoglobin values among the black population can be attributed to nutritional factors and to hereditary anemia affecting only a subset of blacks.

It is well known that the U.S. black population, as a whole, has a lower socioeconomic status than the white population. The correlation of increased nutritional anemia and lower socioeconomic status is well known also (5). Therefore, it would be necessary to compare hemoglobin or hematocrit results between both groups while controlling for socioeconomic status and/or nutritional factors. In the U.S., the main nutritional factor to control for would be iron nutritional status (1). In studies in which biochemical tests were used to control for nutritional status, the mean hemoglobin difference between blacks and whites declined to 0.2 to 0.5 g/dl (15,16). Although smaller, this remaining difference in hemoglobin between the two groups was still statistically significant. However, comparison of the hemoglobin distribution between the two groups found that the hemoglobin distribution of blacks was skewed at the lower hemoglobin end (Fig. 6) (12,17). There was a marked difference in the relationship between the two curves. The skewed hemoglobin distribution did not represent a generalized shift of the entire distribution, but rather a downward skewing of the black distribution. This relationship suggests that a subset of blacks have mild anemia, a factor that would pull the mean hemoglobin downward. Such a finding is compatible with the high prevalence of mild hereditary anemia among blacks, such as α- or β-thalassemia traits (16,18,19).

Although there has been no study that fully excluded all individuals with nutritional deficiency and mild hereditary anemia before the hemoglobin distribution between blacks and whites was compared, the existing evidence suggests that the lower hemoglobin values observed in the black population are probably not the result of normal variation. Therefore, unless there is further evidence to the contrary, it would be prudent not to use a lower hemoglobin cutoff value to define anemia among blacks. If a lower cutoff value were used, both iron deficiency anemia and mild hereditary anemia

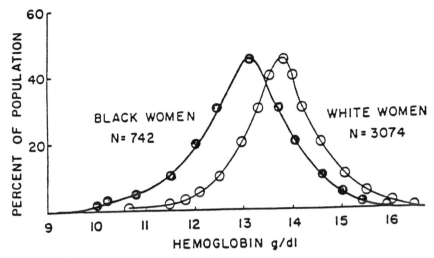

FIG. 6. Examples of hemoglobin distribution among white and black women, aged 18–44 years. Based on data from the NHANES I (17). (Reproduced from ref. 12 with permission by the Johns Hopkins University School of Hygiene and Public Health, © 1979.)

would less likely be detected among blacks (i.e., a higher false-negative rate). Although hemoglobin differences have not been extensively studied for other ethnic groups, a comparative study of American Indian and Asian children with white children found their hemoglobin or hematocrit values to be similar (16,20).

PRACTICAL FIELD TESTS FOR ANEMIA AND IRON DEFICIENCY

Unlike the situation in hospital and research settings, the choice of laboratory tests for iron deficiency in outpatient or field settings is limited. Screening for anemia by either hemoglobin or hematocrit is the most common approach used in a field setting. The main limitation of this approach is that it fails to detect those children who have iron deficiency without anemia.

Both hemoglobin and hematocrit tests provide essentially the same information—the presence or absence of anemia. On a theoretical basis, hemoglobin would be a more sensitive test for iron deficiency, because reduction in hemoglobin synthesis precedes the reduction in red cell volume or numbers. However, the errors of most field methods of measuring hemoglobin or hematocrit would likely exceed the theoretical advantage of the test. Of greater importance is the precision and ease of operation of the field instrument. Because an adequate hemoglobin test usually requires more reagent handling and dilution procedures than the spun hematocrit test, hematocrit is a more commonly used test in clinics and public health settings.

A recently developed hemoglobin device that uses the sodium azide method (HemoCue system) appears to offer certain operational advantages over the hematocrit test (21). This system uses a microcuvette coated with dried sodium azide to collect blood and measure hemoglobin. In laboratory comparisons with standard hemoglobin methods, the accuracy and precision of the system were satisfactory (22). This device is portable and can be operated with a battery, making it suitable for field use.

Among the three commonly used biochemical tests (transferrin saturation, serum ferritin, and EP), only the EP test currently appears to have the potential for routine screening in a field setting. A portable hematofluorometer for EP testing has been developed that directly reads the EP fluorescence response of a drop of whole blood, based on a front-face method (22). Unlike the traditional chemical extraction method of EP measurement, which required multiple procedures and was time-consuming, the hematofluorometer requires no sample preparation and a relatively short time (30 sec). This method was developed because EP is the primary screening test for childhood lead poisoning (23), and in the past decade many public health clinics have gained extensive experience in screening for lead poisoning with the hematofluorometer method. Nevertheless, the EP test also appears to be suitable as a screening procedure for iron deficiency because EP has greater sensitivity than hemoglobin or hematocrit in detecting iron deficiency (24,25). In addition, it has been established as a screening tool in a primary care setting (25). In a study of 4,160 children in which low serum ferritin was used to represent iron deficiency, a measurement of EP $\geq$ 35 µg/dl was able to detect 88% of the 278 children with low serum ferritin, whereas measurement for anemia was able to detect only 59% of the 278 children (23). Although EP is not specific to iron deficiency, the ability to detect children at risk for lead poisoning makes it an attractive screening tool for younger children. The main obstacle to its broader use is that existing portable instruments require vigorous quality control to ensure their proper operation. Also, a uniform standardization procedure is lacking, as well as common units to express the results (Table 1). Until most of these issues can be resolved, it is unlikely that EP will be widely used for screening purposes for iron deficiency.

IRON NUTRITIONAL STATUS OF INFANTS AND YOUNG CHILDREN IN THE U.S.

Using the hematological and iron biochemical laboratory criteria developed from the NHANES II sample, the prevalence of anemia for this sample group can be assessed. The application of test cutoffs to a sample in whom the cutoff criteria were developed may seem circular. Had the laboratory criteria been based on the -2 standard deviation value of the unselected sample (test reference), approximately 2.5% of the sample would be expected to fall below the lower 95% limit when such cutoffs were applied to the original sample. However, it would be appropriate to apply the NHANES II laboratory criteria described above, which were based on the test standards (abnormal subjects excluded), to the original reference sample.

Prevalence of Childhood Anemia Based on NHANES II

The prevalence of anemia among younger American children from 1976 to 1980 has been estimated (Table 4) (7). In the 1- to 2-year age group, the prevalence of anemia represented one of the highest prevalence rates among all age and sex groups in the NHANES II sample. Only women aged 20–44 years had comparable prevalence rates (5.8%). The criterion for anemia used here (hemoglobin < 10.7 g/dl) is 0.3 g/dl of hemoglobin lower than the commonly used value of hemoglobin < 11.0 g/dl recommended by the American Academy of Pediatrics (2). Among children 1 to 2 years of age from the NHANES II sample, the prevalence rate would be 15% if hemoglobin of < 11.0 g/dl were used as the cutoff value for determining anemia.

Prevalence of Iron Deficiency Based on the NHANES II Sample

The prevalence of iron deficiency (with or without anemia) based on multiple abnormal tests was determined for the NHANES II sample population (8). Because most younger children did not have serum ferritin test results, only the MCV model (MCV, Fe/TIBC, and EP) was used to assess the iron nutritional status of those 2 years or younger (Table 5). Another method to estimate the prevalence of iron deficiency is the hemoglobin percentile shift method (7,8). It is based on the hemoglobin percentile shift after those individuals with abnormal iron biochemical test results are excluded. Again, like the results for anemia, the prevalence rate of iron deficiency for the youngest children was one of the highest among all age and sex groups in

TABLE 4. *Estimated prevalence of anemia for younger children*[a]

Age (years)	Anemia criteria	Venipuncture only prevalence (%)	Venipuncture + capillary sample prevalence (%)
1–2	Hgb < 10.7 g/dl	5.7	9.5
3–5	Hgb < 10.9 g/dl	3.5	4.8

[a]Based on NHANES II.

the NHANES II sample population. All three methods provided similar estimations of the prevalence of iron deficiency.

Contribution of Iron Deficiency to Childhood Anemia

Iron deficiency is the major cause of childhood anemia in the U.S. The NHANES II sample population represents an opportunity to evaluate the relationship between hematological and iron biochemical test results of a relatively healthy national sample. For example, a comparison of the mean value of iron biochemical tests for both anemic and nonanemic children indicates that anemic children have a strong tendency toward iron deficiency, in contrast to nonanemic children (Table 6) (7).

The relationship between iron deficiency and childhood anemia can also be determined by the intersect between these two conditions (Table 7). Among younger children, 70% of the anemia was caused by iron deficiency. However, anemia can detect only one-third of the iron-deficient cases, and two-thirds of the iron-deficient cases were not anemic. Thus, anemia may not be the best indicator of iron deficiency. A similar comparison for older children showed a less definite relationship between iron deficiency and anemia.

TABLE 5. *Prevalence of iron deficiency based on multiple laboratory tests and hemoglobin percentile shift method[a]*

Age (years)	Prevalence of iron deficiency (%)		
	Hgb percentile shift	MCV model	Ferritin model
1–2	9.2	9.4	—
3–5	3.6	3.9	4.5

[a]MCV model based on MCV, Fe/TIBC, and EP; ferritin model based on serum ferritin, Fe/TIBC, and EP.
A case of iron deficiency is defined as two or more positive tests.

TABLE 6. *Laboratory characteristics of anemic and nonanemic children 1–2 years of age[a]*

Status	n	Fe (μg/dl)	TIBC (μg/dl)	Fe/TIBC (%)	MCV (fl)	EP (μg/dl of RBC)
Anemic	26	57.8[b]	445[b]	13.0[b]	74.9[b]	126.1[b]
Nonanemic	405	81.3	408	20.2	78.6	67.3

[a]Data taken from NHANES II, 1976–1980: ref. 7.
[b]Anemic group statistically different from nonanemic group, $p < 0.01$.

Prevalence of Anemia Among Low-Income Children

Data from the NHANES II Sample

Because of the detailed family income information available in the NHANES II sample, the prevalence of anemia and iron deficiency can be determined for children from different socioeconomic backgrounds. The prevalence of iron deficiency based on the MCV model can be compared for those above the federal poverty level with those children below the federal poverty level (Table 8). The federal poverty level, established annually by the U.S. Department of Agriculture, is based on family size and total income, a guideline used by a number of government assistance programs. These findings indicate that younger children whose families were below the poverty level had three times the risk of having iron deficiency as those whose families were above the poverty level.

TABLE 7. *Relationship between anemia and iron deficiency in children 1 to 2 years of age from NHANES II*

		Iron deficiency		
		Yes	No	Total
Anemic[a]	Yes	7	3	10 (All anemic)
	No	16	129	145
	Total	23 (all iron def.)	132	155

Percentage of iron-deficient subjects also anemic = 7/23 = 33% (sensitivity).
Percentage of anemic subjects also iron deficient = 7/10 = 70% (positive predictive value).
[a]Anemia is defined as Hgb < 10.7 g/dl. Iron deficiency is defined as two or more positive test results for MCV, transferrin saturation, and EP (MCV model).

TABLE 8. *Prevalence of iron deficiency based on the MCV model according to poverty levels[a]*

Age (years)	Prevalence of iron deficiency (%)	
	Above poverty	Below poverty
1–2	6.7	20.6
3–4	2.5	9.7

[a]Data from ref. 8.

Data from the CDC Pediatric Nutrition Surveillance System

In addition, the prevalence of anemia among children in low income families can be estimated from the information provided by the Pediatric Nutrition Surveillance System (PNSS) from the Centers for Disease Control (CDC). This system collects individual hemoglobin and hematocrit results from various public health clinics in 36 states. In 1987, approximately 2 million clinic records were collected, and approximately 90% of these records were from WIC clinics (Special Supplemental Food Program for Women, Infants, and Children). PNSS data were used to assess the prevalence of anemia in 1987 (Table 9). In part, the relatively high prevalence of anemia in the PNSS data can be explained by the lower income of families enrolled in public health programs, as well as by the preference given to enrollment of anemic children in the WIC program. Another potential explanation for the relatively high prevalence of anemia in the PNSS is that laboratory and reporting errors tend to give the benefit of doubt to children enrolled in such programs, a factor that may inflate the prevalence rate somewhat (26). Consequently, interpreting the prevalence of anemia from PNSS data should be done cautiously.

SUMMARY

Defining iron deficiency properly is a necessary prerequisite for the detection of iron deficiency on an individual or on a population basis. The limitations of hematological and iron biochemical tests should be taken into account in interpreting clinical or epidemiological data on iron deficiency. It is also important to distinguish between testing approaches for general screening, for diagnosis of the cause of anemia, and for estimating the prevalence of iron deficiency in a population. Commonly used hemoglobin or hematocrit tests appear to detect only some iron-deficient children, although most cases of anemia in younger children are related to iron deficiency. Moreover, lower income children have a significantly higher prevalence of anemia and iron deficiency than the national average. Special consideration

TABLE 9. *Prevalence of anemia in low income children monitored by the CDC Pediatric Nutrition Surveillance System (PNSS), 1987[a]*

Age (years)	n	Anemia (%)
0.5–2	996,270	15.9
2–5	949,595	18.6
All	1,945,865	17.2

[a]Anemia is defined as Hgb < 11.0 g/dl or Hct < 33% for children 0.5 to 2 years old, and Hgb < 11.3 g/dl or Hct < 35% for children 2 to 5 years old.

should be given to improving the iron nutritional status of lower income infants and children.

REFERENCES

1. Yip, R., Johnson, C., and Dallman, P. R. (1984): Age-related changes in laboratory values used in the diagnosis of anemia and iron deficiency. *Am. J. Clin. Nutr.,* 39:427–436.
2. Committee on Nutrition, American Academy of Pediatrics (1985): Iron deficiency. In: *Pediatric Nutrition Handbook,* 2nd ed., edited by G. R. Forbes and C. W. Woodruff. American Academy of Pediatrics, Elk Grove, IL.
3. Beutler, E. (1988): The common anemia. *JAMA,* 259:2434–2437.
4. Lee, G. R. (1983): The anemia of chronic disease. *Semin. Hematol.* 20:61–80.
5. Yip, R., and Dallman, P. R. (1988): The roles of inflammation and iron deficiency as causes of anemia. *Am. J. Clin. Nutr.,* 48:1295–1300.
6. Cebul, R. D., Hershey, J. C., and Williams, S. V. (1982): Using multiple tests: series and parallel approaches. *Clin. Lab. Med.,* 2:871–890.
7. Dallman, P. R., Yip, R., and Johnson, C. (1984): Prevalence and causes of anemia in the United States, 1976 to 1980. *Am. J. Clin. Nutr.,* 39:437–445.
8. Expert Scientific Working Group (1984): *Assessment of the Iron Nutrition Status of the U.S. Population Based on Data Collected by the Second National Health and Nutrition Examination Survey, 1976–1980.* Life Science Research Office, Federation of American Society of Experimental Biology, Bethesda, MD.
9. Galen, R. S., and Gambino, S. R. (1975): *Beyond Normality: The Predictive Value and Efficiency of Medical Diagnosis.* John Wiley and Sons, New York.
10. Plan and Operation of the Second National Health and Nutrition Examination Survey, 1976–1980 (1982): *Vital and Health Statistics,* Series 1, no. 232, DHHS Publication No. (PHS) 81–1317, National Center for Health Statistics, Public Health Service. Government Printing Office, Washington, D.C.
11. Ten State Nutrition Survey, 1968–1970. IV. Biochemical. USDHEW publication (HSM) 72–8130. Centers for Disease Control, Atlanta, 1972.
12. Meyers, L. D., Habicht, J. P., and Johnson, C. L. (1979): Components of the difference in hemoglobin concentration in blood between black and white women in the United States. *Am. J. Epidemiol.,* 109:539–549.
13. Garn, S. M., Smith, N. J., and Clark, D. C. (1975): The magnitude and implications of apparent race differences in hemoglobin values. *Am. J. Clin. Nutr.,* 28:563–568.
14. Owen, G. M., and Yanochik-Owen, A. (1977): Should there be a different definition of anemia in black and white children? *Am. J. Public Health,* 67:865–866.
15. Owen, G. M., Lubin, A. H., and Garry, P. J. (1973): Hemoglobin levels according to age, race, and transferrin saturation in pre-school children of comparable socioeconomic status. *J. Pediatr.,* 82:850–851.
16. Yip, R., Schwartz, S., and Deinard, A. S. (1984): Hematocrit values in white, black, and American Indian children with comparable iron status: evidence to support uniform diagnostic criteria for anemia among all races. *Am. J. Dis. Child.,* 138:824–827.
17. Reeves, J. D., Driggers, D. A., Lo, E. Y. T., and Dallman, P. R. (1981): Screening for anemia in infants: evidence in favor of using identical hemoglobin criteria for blacks and Caucasians. *Am. J. Clin. Nutr.,* 34:2154–2157.
18. Johnson, C. S., Tegos, C., and Beutler, E. (1982): Alpha-thalassemia: prevalence and hematologic findings in American blacks. *Arch. Intern. Med.,* 142:1280–1282.
19. Pierce, H. I., Kurachi, S., Sofronniadau, K., and Stamatoyannopoulos, G. (1977): Frequencies of thalassemia in American blacks. *Blood,* 49:981–986.
20. Dallman, P. R., Barr, G. D., Allen, C. M., and Shinefield, H. R. (1978): Hemoglobin concentration in white, black, and Oriental children: is there a need for separate criteria in screening for anemia? *Am. J. Clin. Nutr.,* 31:377–380.
21. Cohen, A. R., and Seidl-Friedman, J. (1988): HemoCue system for hemoglobin measurement: evaluation in anemic and non-anemic children. *Am. J. Clin. Pathol.,* 90:302–305.

22. Blumberg, W. E., Esinger, J., and Lamola, A. A. (1977): The hematofluorometer. *Clin. Chem.,* 23:270–274.
23. Centers for Disease Control (1985): *Prevention of Lead Poisoning in Young Children,* Publication no. 99-2230. Centers for Disease Control, Atlanta.
24. Piomelli, S. (1977): Free erythrocyte porphyrin in the detection of undue absorption of Pb and of Fe deficiency. *Clin. Chem.,* 23:264–269.
25. Yip, R., Schwartz, S., and Deinard, A. S. (1983): Screening for iron deficiency with the erythrocyte protoporphyrin test. *Pediatrics,* 72:214–219.
26. Yip, R., Binkin, N. J., Flashood, L., and Trowbridge, F. L. (1987): Declining prevalence of anemia among low income children in the United States. *JAMA,* 258:1619–1623.

Dietary Iron: Birth to Two Years,
edited by L. J. Filer, Jr.
Raven Press, Ltd., New York © 1989.

The Changing Characteristics of Childhood Iron Nutritional Status in the United States

Ray Yip

Division of Nutrition, Center for Chronic Disease Prevention and Health Promotion, Centers for Disease Control, Atlanta, Georgia 30333

In general, iron deficiency is one of the most common causes of anemia in childhood. For this reason, the prevalence of childhood anemia can be used as an index of childhood iron nutritional status on a population basis.

DECLINING PREVALENCE OF ANEMIA AMONG CHILDREN IN LOW-INCOME HOUSEHOLDS IN THE U.S.

Decline of Anemia Among Children in Low-Income Households

In the past few years, several reports containing evidence of the declining prevalence of anemia among children in low-income households have suggested that their iron nutritional status is improving (1–3). One study, based on children attending a New Haven inner-city public health clinic between 1971 and 1984, found a significant upward shift of hemoglobin distribution between the two time periods (1). The prevalence of anemia (hemoglobin < 9.8 g/dl) among children attending this clinic was 23% in 1971 and 1% in 1984. A similar study based on a single public health clinic in downtown Minneapolis found that the prevalence of childhood anemia was 15% in 1973 and 6% in 1978 (2). The authors of both the New Haven and the Minneapolis studies attributed the improvement in iron nutriture and the resulting decline of anemia to the WIC program (Special Supplemental Food Program for Women, Infants, and Children), which was instituted in the period between the two comparison times of these studies. However, the proposed association of declining anemia with the WIC program requires further examination.

The Pediatric Nutrition Surveillance System (PNSS) of the Centers for Disease Control (CDC) has been collecting hematological data from various public health programs, including the WIC program, since 1975 (3).

Between 1975 and 1986, the annual prevalence of anemia as determined by this surveillance system appeared to be declining, particularly in the late 1970s. However, it is not easy to decide whether this represented a true decline in anemia or whether the apparent decline was caused by a change in the composition of the subjects enrolled in the PNSS. Because the PNSS expanded from five states in 1975 to 36 states in 1988, the influence of a changing population on the system should not be underestimated. To allow for this factor, six states (Arizona, Kentucky, Louisiana, Montana, Oregon, and Tennessee) that had participated in PNSS since 1976 were selected for study of changes in the prevalence of anemia (3). From 1976 to 1985, a total of 1.68 million measurements of hemoglobin and hematocrit were collected from nearly 500,000 children aged 6 months to 5 years in the six selected states (Fig. 1). Overall, 82.3% were from the WIC program, and most of the children enrolled from other programs were also eligible for the WIC program.

The criteria used to define anemia in this study were strict: hemoglobin < 10.3 g/dl or hematocrit < 31% for children aged 6 to 23 months; and hemoglobin < 10.6 g/dl or hematocrit < 32% for children aged 24 to 60 months. Stricter criteria than those commonly used in a clinical setting were applied because of evidence that reporting of hemoglobin and hematocrit measurements was influenced by the WIC program enrollment requirement, i.e., some hemoglobin or hematocrit values near the program cutoff were reported as lower than the observed value (3). To minimize this problem, lower cutoff values likely to be unaffected by reporting practices were used

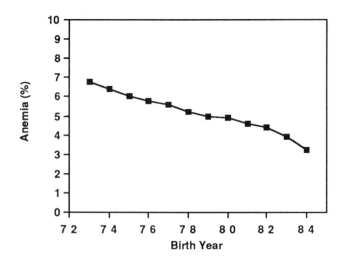

FIG. 1. Prevalence of anemia for each birth-year cohort based on six selected states in the CDC Pediatric Nutrition Surveillance System, 1976–1985. (Reproduced from ref. 3 by permission of *JAMA,* © 1987, American Medical Association.)

to measure trends in the prevalence of anemia. The lower cutoff values resulted in the perception of a lower prevalence of anemia. Therefore, it is important to consider the cutoff values used when the meaning of prevalence rates of anemia is interpreted.

Overall, the prevalence of anemia declined from 6.8% in the initial year to 3.1% in the last birth-year cohort, representing a relative reduction of 54%. Had the hematological data been free from reporting problems, and had the prevalence of anemia been based on a common cutoff value (such as hematocrit < 33% for children under 2 years and hematocrit < 34% for children aged 2–5 years), the estimated prevalence of anemia would have been 18% to 19% for the initial year and 8% to 9% in the last year.

Since previous studies have suggested that the WIC program is a contributing factor in the improvement of infant iron nutrition, the PNSS data offered an opportunity to find such evidence (1,2). PNSS data can be used to compare anemia trends among children based on their program enrollment status as either "non-WIC" or "WIC" children (Fig. 2). The majority of records in this surveillance system are from the WIC program, and the child's WIC enrollment status was collected on records reported to PNSS. A child can be regarded as a non-WIC child at the very first or initial WIC enrollment. Thus, although the record came from a WIC source, the hemoglobin or hematocrit values obtained on the day of WIC enrollment reflected the nutritional status before the child entered the program. A WIC child, on the other hand, has had at least two certifications by the program. Since a typical certification period is 6 months, children with two or more certifica-

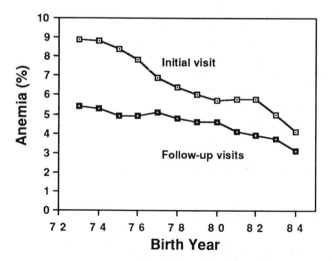

FIG. 2. Comparison of anemia trends of non-WIC and WIC children based on data from the CDC Pediatric Nutrition Surveillance System, 1976–1985. (Reproduced from ref. 3 by permission of *JAMA*, © 1987, American Medical Association.)

tions would have been enrolled in the program for at least 6 months. Similar to the declining trend of the overall group, both WIC and non-WIC groups showed a significant decline in the prevalence of anemia. However, the non-WIC group consistently demonstrated a higher prevalence of anemia than the WIC group throughout the years of the study.

This finding points out two important possibilities. First, WIC children appeared to be nutritionally healthier than non-WIC children, an implication that supports the contention of previous authors that the WIC program may explain the decline in childhood anemia. Second, the prevalence of anemia among non-WIC children also appeared to be declining. It is possible that a generalized improvement of infant and childhood iron nutritional status in the U.S. has contributed to the decline of anemia among non-WIC children. One pitfall in interpreting these comparative data for all WIC and non-WIC children is the lack of comparability of age, i.e., age could have been a confounder. In general, younger children, who have a higher prevalence of anemia or iron deficiency, are more likely to be new enrollees in the WIC program and hence to be classified as non-WIC children. By contrast, older children, who have a lower prevalence of anemia, are more likely to have been in the WIC program for some time and hence to be classified as WIC children. Thus, we also compared age-specific trends of anemia (Fig. 3) (3).

This age-specific comparison demonstrated a similar decline in anemia as well as a higher prevalence of anemia in the non-WIC group than in the WIC group. Since both the WIC program and other public health programs have specific family income criteria for enrollment, it is reasonable to conclude that children in low-income households of the same age who are in the WIC program have a better iron nutritional status than those children from low-income families who are not in the program. However, some may argue that low-income families who join a public program early may differ from those who join a program later or never join at all. Another major factor in the proper interpretation of these declining trends for childhood anemia is whether the sociodemographic composition of WIC enrollment for the six selected states was changing for the better, i.e., more high-risk children enrolled in the earlier years than in the later years. To explore these issues, we used PNSS records from the Tennessee WIC program to examine the influence of sociodemographic factors on anemia trends.

The Influence of Sociodemographic Factors on the Trend of Anemia

Tennessee WIC records were used because they contained key variables on records reported to the CDC PNSS that allowed data linkage with vital birth records from Tennessee (3). Vital birth records contain basic sociodemographic information such as parental age, parental educational level, marital

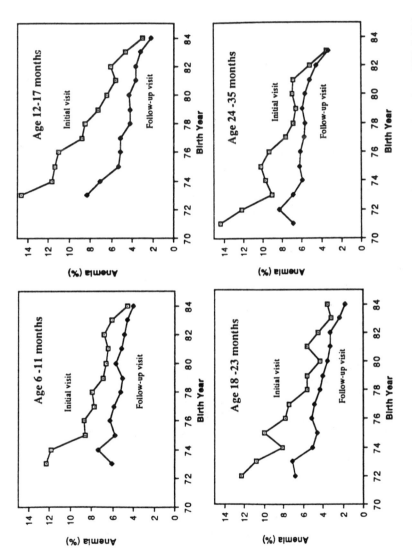

FIG. 3. Age-specific trends in prevalence of anemia. Comparison of WIC (follow-up visit) and non-WIC (initial visit) children based on birth-year cohort. Six selected states from the CDC Pediatric Nutrition Surveillance System, 1976–1985. (Reproduced from ref. 3 by permission of *JAMA*, © 1987, American Medical Association.)

status, and prenatal care patterns. The data linkage procedure added this sociodemographic information to each WIC record for expanded analysis.

From 1975 to 1984, Tennessee-linked WIC birth data contained a total of 319,000 hematocrit measurements from nearly 73,000 children aged 6 to 60 months. A socioeconomic status (SES) scale was developed to characterize each family based on information from birth records. Three risk factors were used to develop the SES scale: (a) mother's age of 17 years or younger at child's birth; (b) mother's education less than 12th grade; and (c) mother unmarried. Low SES was assigned to those children whose families had two or more of the risk factors, intermediate SES to those whose families had only one risk factor, and higher SES to those children whose families had none of the risk factors. The higher SES group was further divided into two subgroups based on whether at least one of the parents had more than a high school education. This division resulted in four SES groups: from high SES (group 1) to low SES (group 4). Tennessee WIC trends in prevalence of anemia were compared for each of the four SES groups to determine whether SES influenced the decline of anemia (Fig. 4). Strict anemia cutoff values were used: hematocrit < 31% for ages 1 to 2 years, and hematocrit < 32% for ages 2 to 5 years (3). From 1975 to 1984, the relative composition of the four SES groups did not improve, although a few more low SES families enrolled in the WIC program in the later years (20% in 1975 and 22% in 1984). Therefore, analysis of the data by SES composition does not support the hypothesis that the improved SES of WIC participants contributed to the declining trend in the prevalence of anemia.

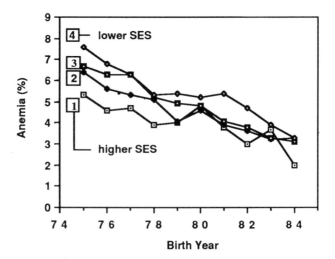

FIG. 4. Comparison of trends in prevalence of anemia for children in four socioeconomic status (SES) groups from the Tennessee WIC program. Group 1 represents high SES and group 4 represents low SES. (Reproduced from ref. 3 by permission of *JAMA*, © 1987, American Medical Association.)

The SES-specific trends for prevalence of anemia in Tennessee indicate that low SES children had the highest prevalence of anemia and high SES children had the lowest prevalence. Over the 10-year period, all four SES groups showed a comparable pattern of decline. Although all WIC children by definition come from lower income backgrounds, there were marked variations in SES and nutritional status within WIC subpopulations (Fig. 4). This information suggests the importance of controlling for SES when the potential health impact of the WIC program is evaluated.

Relationship of the WIC Program to Childhood Iron Nutritional Status

The Tennessee-linked WIC and birth records offered the opportunity to look more closely at the possible influence of participation in the WIC program on childhood iron nutritional status. By using the same approach for the six selected states in determining WIC and non-WIC status, the prevalence of anemia can be compared within each SES group, as defined earlier. Again, the non-WIC children were those who had hematocrit measurements tested upon initial enrollment. Comparisons were made between WIC and non-WIC children for age-specific as well as SES-specific groups (Table 1) (4). Strict cutoff values for anemia were used: hematocrit < 31% for ages 1 to 2 years and hematocrit < 32% for ages 2 to 5 years (3). The information in Table 1 indicates a strong relationship between SES and the prevalence of anemia. However, in each specific SES group, WIC children consistently had a lower prevalence of anemia than non-WIC children. Age-specific groups showed similar patterns. These findings suggest that the WIC program had a positive influence on the iron nutritional status of those enrolled in the program. However, because these comparisons are based on retrospective data, they do not have the power of proof of an appropriately designed prospective study. Nevertheless, these data provide the strongest evidence thus far that the WIC program is associated with reduced childhood anemia and improved childhood iron nutritional status (3,4).

Other Evidence to Support the Improvement of the Iron Nutritional Status of Children in Low-Income Households

Iron Intake Based on the National Food Consumption Survey—
Continuing Survey of Food Intakes by Individuals (CSFII)

The Continuing Survey of Food Intakes by Individuals (CSFII) is a nationwide nutrient intake survey conducted by the U.S. Department of Agriculture. Detailed 1-day nutrient intakes of children 1 to 5 years old were collected in 1977 and 1985 (5). In this survey, low income was defined as 130% of the Federal poverty level, in contrast to the 185% of poverty commonly used for WIC enrollment. The iron intake of children in lower-income households was compared between these two time periods (Table 2). Based upon dietary intake data from the two time periods, infants and children in all income groups had an increase in iron intake, not just the children in low–income households. It is likely that the WIC program contributed to the higher iron intake of infants whose families had low incomes. However, this survey information cannot determine the relative contribution of the WIC program to iron nutrition among children in low-income households.

Comparison of Iron Intake Between WIC and Non-WIC Controls Based on the National WIC Evaluation

The National WIC Evaluation was conducted to assess the effects of the WIC program on pregnant women and children (6). For children, growth, nutrient intake, health care utilization, and psychological development were measured (6). Unfortunately, iron nutritional status was not assessed. The infant and child portion of the study, which was cross-sectional, included 2,619 preschool children whose mothers were also studied. Approximately one-third of the children were currently enrolled in the WIC program, one-

TABLE 1. *Prevalence of anemia of previously enrolled WIC children and newly enrolled non-WIC children aged 6–59 months for four SES groups in the Tennessee WIC Program*

SES group	Prevalence of anemia (%)	
	Non-WIC children	WIC children
1. High SES	3.0	1.9
2.	3.5	2.5
3.	4.1	2.7
4. Low SES	4.2	3.0

TABLE 2. *Comparison of mean iron intake per person per day by income level between Spring 1977 and Spring 1985*

Income level	Age (years)	Daily iron intake (mg)	
		1977	1985
< 130% poverty	1–3	8.7	10.3
	4–5	9.6	11.1
130–300% poverty	1–3	8.2	10.6
	4–5	9.7	10.9
≥ 300% poverty	1–3	8.8	10.6
	4–5	9.8	13.7

third had been enrolled in the past, and one-third had never been enrolled. Nutrient intake data revealed significantly higher iron and vitamin C intake among WIC infants than among non-WIC infants (Table 3) (6). The findings also indicate that infants and children currently enrolled in the WIC program have greater iron and vitamin C intake than those not enrolled. These findings complement the finding of a lower prevalence of anemia among WIC children than among non-WIC children based on the CDC surveillance data and Tennessee WIC data (3).

Summary of the Relationship Between the WIC Program and Improvement in Iron Nutritional Status of Children in Low–Income Households

Thus far, evidence shows a significant reduction of childhood anemia among children in low–income households in the U.S. The best explanation for this decline is the improvement in infant and childhood iron intake. The evidence suggests that WIC enrollment is associated with a lower prevalence of anemia, and the national WIC evaluation report lends further support to this conclusion. Other evidence supporting such a relationship is the WIC food supplementation practice for infants, which provides iron-fortified formula up to 1 year of age for those eligible infants who are not breast fed. It has been well established that iron-fortified formula significantly protects against iron deficiency, in contrast to feeding with non-iron-fortified formula or whole milk (7).

Evidence for a Generalized Improvement in Childhood Iron Nutritional Status in the U.S.

Two additional studies support the finding that the improvement in iron nutritional status and decline in prevalence of anemia are not restricted to children from low-income households (8,9).

TABLE 3. *Comparison of daily mean iron and mean vitamin C intakes for infants and children in the National WIC Evaluation Program*[a]

Nutrients	Age (months)	Current WIC	Past WIC	Controls
Iron (mg)	0–11	21.4	14.3	13.5
	12–59	11.1	9.8	9.9
Vitamin C (mg)	0–11	113.1	98.5	85.7
	12–59	103.9	88.7	92.1

[a]Based on 24-hr dietary recalls.

Declining Prevalence of Anemia in a Middle-Class Setting

If improvement of iron nutrition in infancy and childhood was not restricted to children in low-income households, one would expect that children in middle-class households would show evidence of improvement. To test this hypothesis, a retrospective study was conducted that reviewed hematocrit values from a stable pediatric practice in a middle-class area in Minneapolis from 1969 to 1986 (8). A total of 6,162 hematocrit values were collected from the medical records of 2,432 children; 91% were from well-child visits and 9% were from sick visits. Also collected were 1,846 values of erythrocyte protoporphyrin (EP) measured since 1981 using a portable hematofluorometer. The criteria of anemia for this study were hematocrit < 33% for children under 2 years of age, hematocrit < 34% for children 2 to 5 years old, and hematocrit < 35% for children 6 to 7 years old. An elevated EP value (defined as ≥ 35 µg/dl of whole blood) was used as evidence of iron deficiency (Fig. 5) (9).

Based on these data, several conclusions can be drawn. First, the declining trend of anemia, which is likely the result of improved iron nutrition,

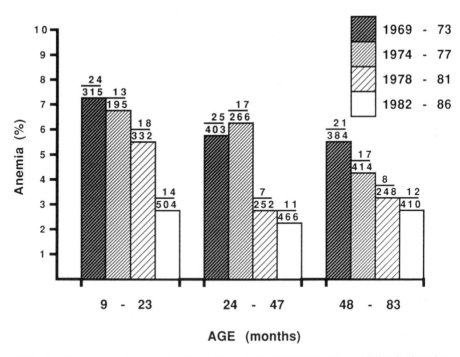

FIG. 5. Prevalence of anemia for three age-specific groups of healthy children for four time periods. The numbers on each bar represent the number of children with anemia (numerator) and all children who had hematocrit measurements (denominator). (Reproduced from ref. 8 by permission of *Pediatrics,* © 1987.)

occurred in a non-low-income setting also. Second, the decline of anemia occurred for younger as well as older children, suggesting that improvement at a younger age may positively influence iron nutritional status in later childhood. Third, in this clinical setting, the prevalence of anemia from 1982 to 1986 was very low: less than 3% of prevalence, the statistical baseline level of a normal population. The low prevalence of anemia in recent years suggests that there is little or no iron deficiency in this study population. The few cases of anemia may represent part of the normal hematocrit distribution, i.e., anemia is defined as the 2.5th percentile of the hematocrit distribution of a healthy sample.

To explore the relationship of anemia and iron deficiency in a setting in which the prevalence of anemia is low, the 1981–1986 hematocrit data from the Minneapolis study were compared with the EP data described above (Table 4). This analysis indicates that more than 90% of the anemic children did not have iron deficiency. These data confirm the suspicion that when the prevalence of anemia is very low, few cases of iron deficiency and iron deficiency anemia are seen. Only 7.4% of those with anemia showed evidence of iron deficiency, based on elevated EP values. Likewise, few of those with iron deficiency were anemic (7.8%). The poor correlation of anemia with iron deficiency indicates that as iron deficiency becomes less frequent, the remaining cases become milder, i.e., without anemia. The implication is that as iron deficiency becomes less common, anemia as a means to detect iron deficiency is less effective. The reduced effectiveness of hemoglobin or hematocrit measurements to detect iron deficiency and the changing epidemiology of iron deficiency suggest the need to reassess the current pediatric practice of screening for iron deficiency.

TABLE 4. *Relationship of anemia and iron deficiency based on elevated erythrocyte protoporphyrin (EP) values of healthy middle-class children attending a private pediatric clinic, 1981–1986[a]*

	Anemia	No anemia	Total
EP ≥ 35 µg/dl, iron deficiency	4 (0.2%)	47 (2.8%)	51[b] (3.0%)
EP < 35 µg/dl, no iron deficiency	50 (3.2%)	1582 (94.0%)	1632 (97.0%)
Total	54[c] (3.2%)	1629 (96.8%)	1683 (100.0%)

[a]Reproduced from ref. 8 with permission from *Pediatrics*, © 1987.
[b]Iron deficient subjects who also have anemia: 4/51 = 7.8%.
[c]Anemic subjects who also have iron deficiency: 4/54 = 7.4%.

Declining Prevalence of Childhood Iron Deficiency in the U.S.

Evidence of declining anemia reported in various studies as well as direct evidence strongly suggest a change in childhood iron nutritional status. Among the biochemical tests performed consistently between the NHANES I, 1970 to 1975, and the NHANES II, 1976 to 1980, were serum iron, total iron binding capacity, and transferrin saturation (10). Because both NHANES surveys were based on national representative samples, and the serum iron and transferrin saturation analyses for both surveys were performed by the same laboratory by the same method, these data can be compared (Fig. 6). The criteria used for defining iron deficiency were transferrin saturation < 9% for children 1 to 2 years of age, < 10% for children 3 to 5 years of age, and < 11% for those 6 years or older. Findings from the two NHANES surveys indicate a significant reduction of childhood iron deficiency from the early 1970s to the late 1970s. Since the NHANES sample is national and not restricted to lower-income families, these findings

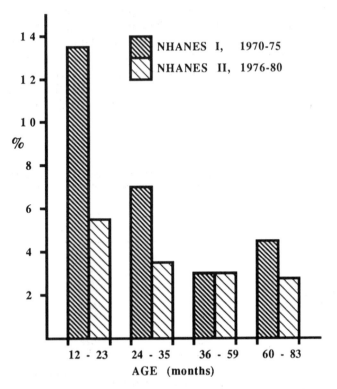

FIG. 6. Comparison of prevalence of childhood iron deficiency, based on low transferrin saturation, between NHANES I, 1970–1975, and NHANES II, 1976–1980.

strengthen the proposition of a generalized improvement of iron nutrition in infancy and childhood.

Evidence to Support a Generalized Improvement in Infant Iron Nutritional Status

Increased iron intake in infancy and childhood is supported by the National Food Consumption Survey (CSFII), which indicated that the increase occurred among all socioeconomic groups (Table 2) (5). The changing pattern of U.S. infant feeding also supports the observed change in iron nutritional status (3,8,11). Infant feeding practices, such as breast feeding, and the use of iron-fortified formula are known to engender better iron nutritional status. On the other hand, infant feeding practices, such as the use of whole milk or non-iron-fortified formula, tend to increase the risk of iron deficiency (7). Several surveys of U.S. infant feeding practices in the past two decades have revealed significant changes: (a) a marked increase in the proportion of breast-fed infants; and (b) the use of iron-fortified formula with a corresponding reduction in the use of whole milk (11–13).

Summary of Improvement of Iron Nutrition in Infancy and Childhood

The changes that have occurred in infant feeding practices can be attributed to the work of a number of dedicated investigators who demonstrated more than two decades ago the deleterious effect of feeding whole milk in infancy and the protective effect of breast feeding and iron-fortified formula against iron deficiency (14–17). These important findings led to public health policy recommendations, education, and promotion of better infant feeding practices (7,18,19). It may be appropriate to view this long road of effort, which resulted in the disappearance of iron deficiency, as a pediatric nutrition success story.

From a public health perspective, an important lesson has also been learned. Better feeding practices have likely resulted in a significant reduction of one of the most common nutritional disorders of children in the U.S. This process can be regarded as another major model of primary prevention in child health care, similar to that of childhood immunization in the prevention and reduction of communicable disease. In general, prevention is a superior approach compared with early screening and treatment, because primary prevention will result in fewer children who become iron-deficient and suffer adverse consequences.

ANEMIA IN CLINICAL PRACTICE: ETIOLOGY AND SCREENING

In this section, two issues will be examined. One issue concerns the significance of other causes of anemia in clinical practice; the other issue concerns a practical approach for screening for iron deficiency when the condition is uncommon.

Major Causes of Anemia in Infancy and Childhood

In a population where iron deficiency anemia is rare, three major causes for anemia need to be considered: (a) technical and statistical anemia (false anemia) (technical anemia is related to laboratory error or lack of accuracy and to errors introduced by capillary sampling; statistical anemia is related to the definition of the normal hemoglobin and hematocrit range and, by definition, 2.5% of a healthy sample is anemic); (b) anemia of infection and inflammation (related to current or recent mild infection and to any condition with an inflammatory response); and (c) mild hereditary anemia (α- and β-thalassemia trait and the mild form of hemoglobinopathies, e.g., hemoglobin E).

Technical and Statistical Anemia

There are two major sources of technical-related errors for hemoglobin and hematocrit measurements: instrument-related and blood-sampling-related. Under the best laboratory circumstances, a small percentage of the results can be inaccurate. When the overall prevalence of anemia is low, the relative role of laboratory errors becomes greater. These errors may be further compounded by the fact that most hemoglobin and hematocrit tests are performed in an outpatient setting, often with less than satisfactory quality control procedures. Capillary blood sampling, the most common method of outpatient pediatric blood sampling, may also introduce another source of error (21,22).

Statistical anemia is related to the fact that the cutoff value of anemia is defined as the -2 standard deviation (2.5th percentile) of the hemoglobin and hematocrit distribution of a healthy population (23). Therefore, by definition, 2.5% of a healthy population with no risk of nutritional or health disorders is classified as anemic. When the prevalence of childhood anemia is low, these cases of "false anemia" can outnumber *bona fide* cases.

Anemia of Mild Infections

A severe inflammatory response as well as severe infection can result in significant anemia (20,24). In the past several years, the role of mild and common childhood infection in causing mild anemia and altered iron metabolism has become better recognized (8,25,26). The prevalence of anemia among well and sick children, based on a study of Minneapolis middle-class children, indicates the important role of current childhood infection in the development of anemia (Fig. 7). The sick children mainly had upper respiratory infections, gastroenteritis, and otitis media. On average, the prevalence of anemia for these children was two to three times that of those who were well (8).

In addition to current infection, recent infection or illness appears to influence the incidence of anemia. A study of 1-year-old infants at Travis Air Force Base demonstrated that the risk of anemia was several times higher in infants who had an infection within a month of the hemoglobin test. Recent infection was associated with evidence of an inflammatory process, based on an elevated erythrocyte sedimentation rate (ESR) (25) (Fig. 8). Since infections such as upper respiratory infection, otitis media, and gastroenteritis are common in early childhood, their role in anemia can be substantial, especially when the prevalence of iron deficiency is low.

Infection or inflammatory events alter most iron biochemical tests in the same direction as iron deficiency, i.e., reduced serum iron, reduced

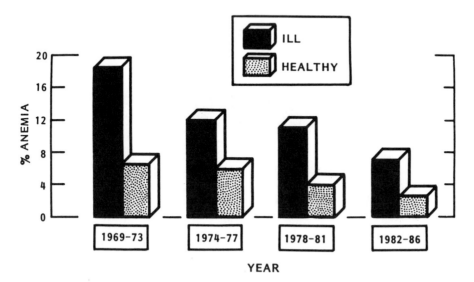

FIG. 7. Comparison of prevalence of anemia among healthy and sick children over four time periods, based on data from a middle-class pediatric practice in Minneapolis. (Reproduced from ref. 8 by permission of *Pediatrics,* © 1987.)

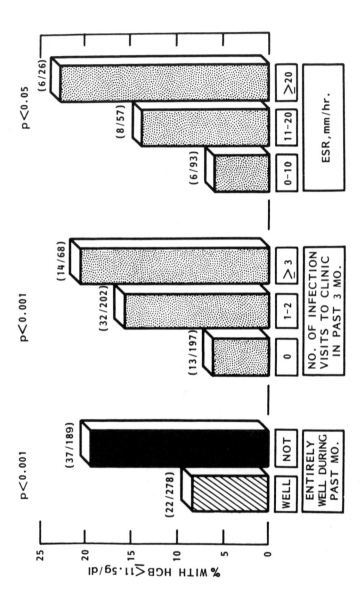

FIG. 8. Prevalence of anemia and low normal hemoglobin (< 11.5 g/dl) in relation to prior illness or infection and to ESR. Significance of difference between groups estimated by χ^2 tests. Number in brackets indicates number of infants with hemoglobin < 11.5 g/dl over total in each group. (Reproduced from ref. 25 by permission of the C.V. Mosby Co., © 1984.)

transferrin saturation, and elevated EP (24). The impact of recent infection on iron biochemical tests is shown in Table 5 (25). Comparisons were based on the number of infection-related visits to a clinic over a 3-month period. Because serum ferritin can become elevated during an inflammatory process, opposite to its direction in iron deficiency (25), it is helpful in differentiating anemia related to iron deficiency from infection or inflammation. Because of the strong influence of the inflammatory process on iron metabolism, appropriate laboratory evaluation for iron nutritional status needs to be conducted when a child is free from recent and current infection.

Mild Hereditary Anemia

Among the common forms of "mild hereditary anemia," thalassemia is the most important one (20). The thalassemias represent a diverse group of inherited anemias that are related to a variety of defects of globin chain synthesis and manifest themselves as various degrees of microcytic anemia. Based on the specific globin synthetic defect, the two most common forms are α-thalassemia and β-thalassemia. The homozygous form of thalassemia, also known as thalassemia major, represents the rare but severe form of anemia. The heterozygous form of thalassemia, also known as thalassemia minor or thalassemia trait, represents the more common but mild form of anemia. This latter form of thalassemia, which is relatively common in certain subpopulations, presents a challenge in the differential diagnosis of iron deficiency anemia. Thalassemia is more common among individuals of African, Middle Eastern, and Asian extraction. Among the American black population, the estimated prevalence of β-thalassemia trait ranges from 1.4% to 3.5%, and the prevalence of α-thalassemia trait ranges from 5.7% to 7.0% (27,28). On average, either type of thalassemia can reduce hemoglobin by 0.5–1 g/dl. While a shift of 0.5 g/dl of hemoglobin may not seem significant in an individual, a generalized downshift of 0.5 g/dl of hemoglobin for a normal population will increase the baseline prevalence of anemia

TABLE 5. *Comparison of laboratory findings related to iron nutrition for sick and well 1-year-old infants[a]*

No. of visits	n	Hgb (g/dl)	MCV (fl)	EP (µg/dl)	Fe/TIBC (%)	Ferritin (µg/l)
0	197	12.7	78.1	79.4	20.5	22.1
1–2	202	12.4	77.1	85.7	19.4	25.0
≥3	68	12.3	76.4	93.3	17.6	27.6
ANOVA *p*		0.005	0.05	0.01	0.2	0.07

[a]Data from infant iron nutrition study of Air Force personnel at Travis Air Force Base, California. Reproduced from ref. 25.

from 2.5% to 6.9% if the shift is 0.5 g/dl, and increase the prevalence of anemia to 16.0% if the shift is 1 g/dl. Therefore, this form of mild anemia can play an important role in contributing to the prevalence of anemia (22,27,28). It is likely that the "load" of thalassemia traits among blacks is responsible for a mild but significant reduction of mean hemoglobin in comparison with whites.

Anemia that does not respond to oral iron treatment requires further evaluation, such as red cell indices determined by an electronic blood counter; this evaluation may be helpful in differentiating thalassemia trait from iron deficiency. Also, iron-related tests such as serum ferritin or EP can be used to determine the presence of iron deficiency. Although microcytic anemia related to iron deficiency usually has a significantly elevated EP level, microcytic anemia related to thalassemia trait will have a normal or mildly elevated EP value (29).

Clinical and Public Health Directions

There are still high-risk subpopulations in the U.S., such as lower–income families, whose children have a much higher prevalence of iron deficiency. Both educational and nutritional support services such as WIC may need to be expanded and targeted toward these high-risk infants and children. Another unresolved issue is whether iron-fortified formula given during the 6th to 12th months of life affects later iron nutritional status. Significant conflicts exist between existing recommendations and existing scientific data (30). A proper evaluation of this issue, particularly among lower income infants, may resolve these differences.

Based on these observations, the following recommendations can be made (31,32): (a) In areas where childhood iron deficiency is still high, such as developing countries, hemoglobin and hematocrit measurements are the primary tool for detecting iron deficiency. (b) In the U.S., particularly in middle-class settings, where childhood iron deficiency is relatively low, the limitation of using anemia to detect iron deficiency should be recognized as well as the need to consider other common causes of anemia such as infection and thalassemia trait. Screening for anemia should be performed when a child is free from current or recent illness, and evaluation for thalassemia should be considered for those who fail to respond to iron therapy.

In addition, if the prevalence of anemia is very low, i.e., less than 2–3%, discontinuation of routine anemia screening should be considered. Instead, selective evaluation should be performed for those children with significant medical or nutritional risk factors for anemia, such as premature birth, and early or excessive use of whole milk.

Finally, the EP test can be considered as the screening test for iron deficiency instead of hemoglobin or hematocrit measurements. The EP test is more sensitive and specific for detection of iron deficiency than anemia screening (9). In addition, it can potentially detect those children with lead toxicity, thus enhancing its usefulness as a child health screening tool.

SUMMARY

It is evident that significant reductions in childhood anemia have occurred in the U.S., which are likely related to the improvement of iron nutrition in infancy and childhood. Improved iron nutritional status undoubtedly is the result of changing infant feeding practices in the U.S., such as increased breast feeding, increased usage of iron-fortified infant formula, and reduced consumption of whole milk in infancy. For children in lower-income households, the WIC program appears to have played a role in the improvement of iron nutrition by providing supplemental food high in iron content during infancy. The improvement of childhood iron nutrition not only reduced the prevalence of childhood anemia, but the nature of the remaining cases of anemia also changed, i.e., more cases of anemia were related to causes other than iron deficiency. The changing pattern of childhood anemia will require the reassessment of existing clinical procedures for screening and diagnosis of iron deficiency in childhood.

ACKNOWLEDGMENT

The author thanks Dr. Peter R. Dallman and Dr. Nancy J. Binkin for their review and helpful comments.

REFERENCES

1. Vazquez-Seoane, P., Windom, R., and Pearson, H. A. (1985): Disappearance of iron deficiency anemia in a high risk infant population given supplemental iron. *N. Engl. J. Med.*, 313:1239–1240.
2. Miller, V., Swaney, S., and Deinard, A. S. (1985): Impact of the WIC program on the iron status of infants. *Pediatrics*, 75:100–105.
3. Yip, R., Binkin, N. J., Flashood, L., and Trowbridge, F. L. (1987): Declining prevalence of anemia among low income children in the United States. *JAMA*, 258:1619–1623.
4. Yip, R., Binkin, N. J., Flashood, L., and Trowbridge, F. L. (1987): Does WIC improve the health outcomes of low income children? An evaluation based on Tennessee-linked WIC and birth data. *Am. J. Clin. Nutr.*, 45:841.
5. Human Nutrition Information Service (1985): National Food Consumption Survey: continuing survey of food intakes by individuals: women 19–50 years and their children 1–5 years, 1 day, 1985. U.S. Dept. of Agriculture, CSFII Report 85-1.
6. Rush, D., Leighton, J. L., Sloan, N. L., et al. (1988): The national WIC evaluation. VI. Study of infants and children. *Am. J. Clin. Nutr.*, 48:484–511.
7. Committee on Nutrition, American Academy of Pediatrics (1976): Iron supplementation for infants. *Pediatrics*, 58:765–768.
8. Yip, R., Walsh, K. M., Goldfarb, M. G., and Binkin, N. J. (1987): Declining prevalence of anemia in childhood in a middle-class setting: a pediatric success story? *Pediatrics*, 80:330–334.

9. Yip, R., Schwartz, S., and Deinard, A. S. (1983): Screening for iron deficiency with the erythrocyte protoporphyrin test. *Pediatrics*, 72:214–219.
10. Yip, R., Binkin, N. J., and Trowbridge, F. L. (1986): Declining childhood anemia prevalence in the U.S.: evidence of improving iron nutrition. *Blood*, 68:51a.
11. Martinez, G. A., and Nalezienski, J. P. (1979): The recent trend in breast feeding. *Pediatrics*, 64:686–692.
12. Sarett, H. P., Bain, K. R., and O'Leary, J. C. (1983): Decision on breast feeding or formula feeding and trends in infant feeding practice. *Am. J. Dis. Child.*, 137:719–725.
13. Fomon, S. J. (1987): Reflections on infant feeding in the 1970s and 1980s. *Am. J. Clin. Nutr.*, 46:171–182.
14. MacKay, H. M. M. (1931): Anemia in infancy with special reference to iron deficiency. Medical Research Council Special Report, Series No. 157.
15. Anyon, C. P., and Clarkson, K. G. (1974): Cow's milk, a cause of iron deficiency anemia in infants. *N.Z. Med. J.*, 74:24.
16. Andelman, M. B., and Sered, B. (1966). Utilization of dietary iron by term infants. *Am. J. Dis. Child.*, 111:45.
17. Gross, S., Vergis, M., and Good, A. (1968): The relationship between milk protein and iron content on hematologic values in infancy. *J. Pediatr.*, 73:521.
18. Committee on Nutrition, American Academy of Pediatrics (1969): Iron balance and requirements in infancy. *Pediatrics*, 43:134.
19. Committee on Nutrition, American Academy of Pediatrics (1971): Iron fortified formula. *Pediatrics*, 47:786.
20. Beutler, E. (1988): The common anemia. *J.A.M.A.*, 259:2434–2437.
21. Thomas, W. J., and Collins, T. M. (1982): Comparison of venipuncture blood counts with microcapillary measurements in screening for anemia in one-year-old infants. *J. Pediatr.*, 101:32–35.
22. Young, P. C., Hamill, B., Wasserman, R. C., and Dickerman, J. D. (1986): Evaluation of capillary microhematocrit as a screening test for anemia in pediatric office practice. *Pediatrics*, 78:206–209.
23. Galen, R. S., and Gambino, S. R. (1975): *Beyond Normality: The Predictive Value and Efficiency of Medical Diagnosis*. John Wiley and Sons, New York.
24. Lee, G. R. (1983): The anemia of chronic disease. *Semin. Hematol.*, 20:61–80.
25. Reeves, J. D., Yip, R., Kiley, V. A., and Dallman, P. R. (1984): Iron deficiency in infancy: the influence of mild antecedent infection. *J. Pediatr.*, 105:874–879.
26. Jansson, L. T., Kling, S., and Dallman, P. R. (1986): Anemia in children with acute infections seen in a primary pediatric outpatient clinic. *Pediatr. Infect. Dis.*, 5:424.
27. Johnson, C. S., Tegos, C., and Beutler, E. (1982): Alpha-thalassemia: prevalence and hematologic findings in American blacks. *Arch. Intern. Med.*, 142:1280–1282.
28. Pierce, H. I., Kurachi, S., Sofronniadau, K., and Stamatoyannopoulos, G. (1977): Frequencies of thalassemia in American blacks. *Blood*, 49:981–986.
29. Stockman, J. A., Weiner, L. S., Simon, G. E., Stuart, M. J., and Oski, F. A. (1975): The measurement of free erythrocyte porphyrin (FEP) as a simple means of distinguishing iron deficiency from beta-thalassemia trait in subjects with microcytosis. *J. Lab. Clin. Med.*, 85:113–119.
30. Tunnessen, W. W., and Oski, F. A. (1987): Consequences of starting whole cow milk at six months of age. *J. Pediatr.*, 111:813–816.
31. Dallman, P. R. (1987): Has routine screening of infants for anemia become obsolete in the United States? *Pediatrics*, 80:439–441.
32. Dallman, P. R., and Yip, R. (1989): Changing characteristics of childhood anemia. *J. Pediatr.*, 114:161–164.

Dietary Iron: Birth to Two Years,
edited by L. J. Filer, Jr.
Raven Press, Ltd., New York © 1989.

Discussion

Dr. Walter: Exactly what do you mean by the ferritin model? When it is determined that a person is anemic or iron-deficient on the basis of the ferritin model, does that mean that all three tests must be abnormal?

Dr. Yip: No, two or more.

Dr. Walter: Two or more, including ferritin?

Dr. Yip: No. In the published studies from the second National Nutrition and Health Examination Survey, the ferritin model uses three tests; if two or more of those three tests are positive, this identifies a case of iron deficiency. If ferritin results are not available, and MCV is substituted for ferritin and if two of the three tests are positive, this also defines a case of iron deficiency.

Dr. Walter: What is the extent of overlap? How many have low transferrin saturation and positive EP (erythrocyte protoporphyrin) results?

Dr. Yip: Overlap varies from one age group to another. In younger children, about 50% of the positive EP cases will also have low ferritin levels. Also 50% of the positive EP cases overlap with those having low transferrin saturation. Thus, each test overlaps with any other test by only 50%.

Dr. Walter: Are the tests done simultaneously?

Dr. Yip: Basically, one has the three test results at the same time, and if two of the three results are positive or three of three are positive, it is a case of iron deficiency. It is unfortunate that the terms, MCV model and ferritin model, have been used in the literature without much of a description of the genesis of the concept of multiple testing. There has been little discussion of the reasons for the need to use multiple testing to define iron deficiency.

Dr. Dallman: It was just a historical accident that the two models were used in the first place. When NHANES was carried out, ferritin measurement was a new test. Thus, it was only determined in about 20% to 25% of the population. So, if one wanted to use the entire population studied in NHANES, approximately 18,000 people, one was forced to use the MCV model. If the ferritin model was used, one could only analyze the data from about 20% to 30% of the population.

Dr. Filer: How much can you change data overlap by changing the cutoff points for each test?

Dr. Yip: Unfortunately, for each test the cutoff point is a floating value. Some investigators use cutoff points for ferritin of less than 15 µg/liter; others use less than 12 µg/liter and some use less than 10 µg/liter. Some use age-specific or categorical cutoff points.

Dr. Owen: In NHANES II, was the group of persons for whom there were ferritin levels a random sample, or were these individuals who had hemoglobin values below 7 g/dl?

Dr. Yip: In the original sampling strategy, serum ferritin measurements were scheduled for 10% of all of the study population. Persons with certain abnormal hematologic and other abnormal iron tests were to constitute another 10%. Because of methodological problems, the sample size was expanded by another 10% to 15%. Analysis of the ferritin data from NHANES II turned out to be a problem because the tests were carried out at several different times and for different technical or sampling reasons.

Dr. Oski: Are the data that you presented from the NHANES II study "color-blind?"

Dr. Yip: The sample is a U.S. probability sample. Therefore, Black and Hispanic populations are included. Due to experimental design, the actual sampling procedure oversampled minority groups and lower-income areas to obtain ethnic-specific information. When we analyze the data, however, we statistically remodel it to fit a true sample of the U.S. Thus, the data are weighted according to the U.S. demographics and are "color-blind."

Dr. Owen: Are you going to account for hereditary anemia in NHANES III?

Dr. Yip: Unfortunately, the hematological component of NHANES III has been grossly shortchanged, compared with the other components programmed for this survey. Survey planners were unable to identify a strong laboratory hematologist willing to participate as a consultant to the government or be the principal person in charge of this survey component. The iron profile is just one part of a large biochemical component. As requests for different tests come in, more and more things are cut out, including part of the hematological testing. Testing may be limited to a CBC. Serum samples will be frozen for future analyses; however, whole blood is not to be saved.

Dr. Filer: Dr. Oski, would you like to comment on the effects of race?

Dr. Oski: In our own experience, when we have excluded known variables, we have not been able to demonstrate a difference between blacks and whites with respect to hemoglobin values.

Dr. Dallman: I am undecided on this issue. In NHANES II, the difference in hemoglobin level between black and white adult males who have virtually no iron deficiency, was over 1 g. From these data we cannot distinguish those who have thalassemia syndromes from those who don't, but the curves were very, very close to being completely shifted over, rather than skewed in one direction. Therefore, if one only considers adult males and applies standard hematologic criteria, many of the black adult males would be defined as iron-deficient. Black females, in contrast, had a higher prevalence of iron deficiency by whatever measure one elected to use. Thus, one can argue that even if there is a discrepancy in the hemoglobin cutoff point, by using the same point for blacks and whites, one is catching more of that zone of overlap and from a policy perspective, one can justify the use of one point. These are the two sides of the argument and I am really undecided. I think it depends on which population we are talking about. If somebody said that we have a tremendous problem with black adult males, then I would say that the premise is false and the criteria should be reexamined.

Dr. Yip: I agree with Dr. Dallman that there are no data for black males indicating that they are iron-deficient. My current plan is to go back to the data from NHANES done in the early 1970s because it provided data on the erythrocyte sedimentation rate (ESR) which was never measured later. It is an indicator of inflammation and disease status and a strong predictor of anemia. When there is a slightly elevated ESR, the hemoglobin level will be coming down. Dr. Dallman and I did a study last year to characterize the impact of mild inflammation on anemia. Even in the 40- to 50-years-plus age groups, more blacks were affected by some type of inflammatory process that can be documented in the laboratory by ESR than were identified by medical history. I am thinking of focusing the analysis of NHANES I data on persons 18 to 40 years of age and excluding those older persons who have more inflammatory conditions or increased ESRs.

Dr. Owen: Are you saying that the blacks studied in NHANES I had higher ESRs, excluding individuals who were anemic?

Dr. Yip: No. There are two phenomena. If one is either from a lower socioeconomic status or black, one is more likely to have a higher ESR. These two factors seem to go together. Generally, people who have significantly higher ESRs have significantly lower hemoglobin values.

Dr. Yip: At the present, the evidence we have is against separate criteria for blacks and whites, but a more definitive study should be done.

Dr. Filer: Are the same racial differences present in infants and children?

Dr. Yip: There have been several studies from the Washington, D.C. area that have examined black populations without a white control group. These investigators have characterized the distribution curves and were able to show the presence of a subpopulation that is significantly skewing the data. Studies from Howard University, which excluded infants and children with iron deficiency, support the possibility that a subpopulation of blacks is dragging down the average for the entire group. This observation does not support the idea that every black person has a hemoglobin level that is 0.5 g less than what would be expected from a normal distribution.

Dr. Dallman: I would like to clarify my earlier comments. What I am undecided about is not whether to use separate criteria, because using separate criteria creates many problems. What I think is important, though, is to examine how uniform criteria are used because the interpretations for the adult black population are simply wrong. I think one has to scrutinize more carefully how uniform criteria are being used.

Dr. Yip: If separate criteria are adopted because some people have hereditary anemia and the cutoff point is lower, these separate criteria may later fail to identify black children who are at the same level of nutritional risk as white children. Thus, adopting these separate criteria is an important undertaking requiring careful consideration.

Dr. Oski: You showed the correlation between EP and ferritin. Would you get the same relationship between EP and serum iron?

Dr. Yip: Yes.

Dr. Owen: What was the number of children in the 1- to 2-year age group in NHANES II?

Dr. Yip: There were 155 who had complete iron testing with venous blood. The combined group numbered 350, if those with capillary blood sampling were included.

Dr. Walravens: Did you say that in order to participate in the WIC Program, hematocrits should be done every 6 months? I fill out many WIC forms and we do one hematocrit every 5 years.

Dr. Yip: There are differences because many local WIC programs have their own local requirements. The most liberal programs that I know of will waive the second measurement if the hematocrit was measured 6 months before. In the majority of WIC programs (those that are actually run by Public Health Clinics), such measurements will be done every 6 months, which, in a sense, almost seems to be an excessive use of resources.

Dr. Filer: Did you eliminate the data from low-birth-weight infants from the calculation comparing the initial visit and follow-up visit groups?

Dr. Yip: No. They were not eliminated in this portion of the analysis.

Dr. Walter: You said that the age group of 12 to 17 months is at the highest risk for iron deficiency. According to our data, the 6- to 11-months age group has a higher risk.

Dr. Yip: In the U.S., the age of highest risk for iron deficiency is 15 months.

Dr. Filer: I agree. Historically, that has been the finding in the U.S.

Dr. Yip: Dr. Owen, do you have any explanation for why American Indian children have a lower prevalence of anemia?

Dr. Owen: I don't think that it is due to altitude. However, when Stanley Garn examined the preschool and 10-State Survey data and subdivided it on the basis of relative fatness (weight for height and skin folds), he found that greater weight for height was associated with higher hemoglobin concentrations.

Dr. Oski: Do the American Indians breast-feed for longer periods of time?

Dr. Yip: I do not know. I would like to do a follow-up study to contrast the Arizona Navajo and Hopi populations with the urban Indian, white, and Hispanic populations. We are interested in assessing nutrition feeding practices as well as the hematological data. If the lower prevalence of anemia among the Indian is a true phenomenon, we might be able to learn something about positive infant feeding patterns that can be recommended and stressed in health promotion education. Unfortunately, we are always chasing after problems and the follow-up of positive findings tends to have a lower priority.

Dr. Yip: All of our data including those on Indian infants and children are adjusted for altitude. We automatically subtract a small amount of hemoglobin for children who live over 4,000 feet. We have very few data on children who live at altitudes greater than 8,000 feet.

Dr. Ziegler: Dr. Owen, you suggested that fatness might be the explanation for higher hemoglobin values in the Hopi and Navajo. Does fatness begin to show up in infancy and early childhood?

Dr. Owen: Yes. These children are heavier for their lengths or heights.

Dr. Yip: We have considerable surveillance data on Indian subpopulations, and the average weight for heights for these populations is definitely greater than that for other low-income populations.

Dr. Walravens: What is the cutoff value in your MCV model?

Dr. Yip: For younger infants and children it is probably 71 fl.

Dr. Walravens: It is 80 fl in your illustration.

Dr. Yip: No. That is different. That is the MCV model criteria specific for determining who is iron-deficient. We are willing to be more generous in that particular approach to identify more people who have questionable status. The distribution doesn't actually shift very much.

Dr. Filer: A crucial issue our Congress faces at the present time is whether the WIC program is worth the large sums of money spent on it. I don't think the David Rush study convinced many people that it is a good program. The Tennessee study that you presented today shows me, for the first time, the real reasons why the WIC program is doing what it should do. I am very pleased that you are presenting the study to our group because these are unpublished data directly from the computer.

Dietary Iron: Birth to Two Years,
edited by L. J. Filer, Jr.
Raven Press, Ltd., New York © 1989.

The Causes of Iron Deficiency in Infancy

Frank A. Oski

*Department of Pediatrics, Johns Hopkins University School of Medicine, Baltimore,
Maryland 21205*

Iron deficiency in infants is the result of an imbalance between the sum of an infant's endowment at birth and subsequent intake and the sum of the infant's needs for growth and the replacement of losses, both normal and abnormal. Although all of these factors may contribute to iron deficiency, rapid growth in association with a lack of adequate dietary iron appear to be the primary factors.

IRON ENDOWMENT AT BIRTH: RELATION TO MATERNAL STORES

The iron content of the newborn infant is approximately 75 mg/kg of body weight, as determined by carcass analysis of stillbirths (1–3). Studies performed during pregnancy indicate that the iron content and the weight of the fetus increase proportionally with age (Fig. 1) (4); thus, throughout gestation, the fetus tends to maintain a constant iron content of about 75 mg/kg (4).

In the fetus, iron is present in three forms: hemoglobin iron, tissue iron, and storage iron. The bulk of the iron endowment, approximately 66%, is in the form of hemoglobin iron. One gram of hemoglobin contains 3.4 mg of elemental iron. An infant weighing 3 kg with a blood volume of approximately 270 ml and a hemoglobin concentration of 17 g/dl would have 156 mg of iron present in the circulating red cell mass, from a total body iron of 225 mg.

The fetus receives its iron indirectly from the maternal circulation, where it is transported against a concentration gradient rapidly and unidirectionally from mother to fetus across the placenta (4). Maternal iron is transported to the placenta bound to transferrin, which gives up its iron to transferrin receptors located on the placental microvillus membrane (5). The iron is then transported through the placenta and becomes associated with transferrin in the fetal circulation.

Controversy continues about the role of maternal iron deficiency in the iron endowment of the fetus. Most data indicate that the hemoglobin concentration in the cord blood of infants born to anemic, iron-deficient mothers does not differ from that of infants born to iron-sufficient mothers (6–8). However, it has been observed that the red cell volume and total hemoglobin mass are significantly reduced in infants born to anemic, iron-deficient mothers even though the hemoglobin concentration in the cord blood is unaffected (9). In addition, Singla and co-workers (10) observed sharply reduced cord blood hemoglobin values in infants born to very anemic mothers. In mothers with a hemoglobin value of less than 6.0 g/dl, the mean hemoglobin concentration in their infants was 12.7 g, in contrast to 18.7 g in infants born to mothers whose hemoglobin values were greater than 11.0 g/dl at the time of delivery.

Most investigators have been unable to demonstrate any relationships

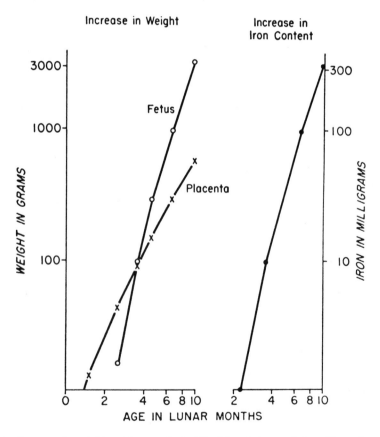

FIG 1. Increase in weight and iron content of the fetus during gestation. (Reproduced from ref. 4 by permission of the University of California Press, © 1958.)

between maternal and infant serum ferritin concentrations (11,12), while others have reported that both the mean weight and the geometric mean of the serum ferritin concentration of neonates of iron-deficient mothers were significantly lower than those of mothers with "normal" iron stores (13). Of interest is the observation (14) that cord blood erythrocyte protoporphyrin, not serum ferritin, may be an index of maternal iron status in the last trimester and that maternal free erythrocyte protoporphyrin in the last trimester predicts the magnitude of the decline in the infant's hemoglobin value measured at 6 weeks of age.

At present, although iron deficiency is very common in mothers during the latter half of pregnancy, there is little compelling evidence that this anemia, unless unusually severe, affects the frequency of iron deficiency in their infants during the first 2 years of life. Far more important to the infant's iron endowment are birth weight and the increase or decrease in the hemoglobin mass at birth, caused by early or late cord clamping, perinatal blood loss, and the occurrence of fetal to maternal hemorrhage.

IRON NEEDS DURING INFANCY

In the normal full-term infant, iron stores are adequate to maintain a state of iron sufficiency for approximately 4 months of growth, whereas in the premature infant, iron stores may become inadequate much earlier, depending on the infant's birth weight, rate of growth, and transfusion history (15).

The infant's iron intake must supplement the iron endowment in order to meet the needs for growth and to replace normal losses. Normal iron losses from the body are small and relatively constant except during episodes of diarrheal disease when they may increase. About two-thirds of iron losses occur from the extrusion of cells from the intestinal mucosa and the remainder from desquamated cells of the skin and urinary tract. In the normal infant, these losses average approximately 20 µg/kg/day [based on published data (6)].

Iron requirements for growth can be approximated. If one calculates the iron requirements of a hypothetical infant who weighs 3 kg at birth and 10 kg at 1 year of age, such an infant may require as much as 270 mg of additional iron during the first year of life (Table 1). This requirement would be maximal, indicating a need to absorb and incorporate approximately 0.7 mg of iron per day. Such an intake would not only prevent the development of iron deficiency anemia but would maintain normal body iron stores as well. Based on such calculations, it has been recommended (16) that the iron intake of term infants should be 1 mg/kg/day, beginning no later than 4 months of age, and the intake of preterm infants should be 2 mg/kg/day, beginning no later than 2 months of age.

Nutritional iron deficiency in term infants begins to appear only after the iron endowment has been depleted. This depletion normally occurs after 6 months of age in a child with the usual growth rate. When iron deficiency is observed before the infant's birth weight has increased by 200% to 250%, one should suspect that the infant was born with a subnormal iron endowment or has experienced unusual blood losses.

PREVALENCE OF IRON DEFICIENCY: IMPACT OF SOCIOECONOMIC STATUS

The prevalence of iron deficiency varies widely depending on the criteria employed to establish the diagnosis. Variables include age and socioeconomic status of the patients surveyed, the extent of the population's participation in the Special Supplemental Food Program for Women, Infants, and Children (WIC), the prevalence and duration of human milk feeding, the age at which whole cow's milk was introduced into the diet, and the extent and duration of the feeding of iron-fortified infant formulas or iron-enriched infant cereals.

As a result of apparent changes in infant feeding patterns that appear to have produced changes in the prevalence of iron deficiency anemia, comparisons of the prevalence of iron deficiency by decade are difficult to interpret. However, a study comparing prevalence of anemia (hemoglobin < 11 g/dl) and iron deficiency (transferrin saturation < 10%) among children in a relatively low-income population with those in a higher-income population suggests that socioeconomic status is a factor in the genesis of iron deficiency. Studies performed in 1979 to 1980 indicated that 30% of infants seen in a U.S. Public Health Service clinic (17) were anemic and approximately 25% were iron-deficient (18), compared with 8% who were found to be anemic and 11% who were iron-deficient in a private practice (19).

TABLE 1. *Iron requirements during the first year of life in a hypothetical infant*

Age	Birth	1 year
Weight (kg)	3	10
Hemoglobin (g/100 ml)	17.0	11.0
Blood volume (ml/kg)	90.0	75.0
Total blood volume (ml)	270.0	750.0
Total body hemoglobin (g)	47.9	82.5
Hemoglobin iron (mg)	162.8	280.5
Tissue iron (7 mg/kg)	21.0	70.0
Storage iron (10 mg/kg)	30.0	100.0
Total body iron	213.8	450.0
Total yearly iron losses (20 µg/kg/day)		47.0
Exogenous iron requirement (mg)		283
Daily iron requirement (mg)		0.78

Two recently published studies have reported an improvement in the iron status of children from low-income families (20,21) and a decline in the prevalence of anemia during the past 15 years. These authors suggested that participation in the WIC program is the factor primarily responsible for the observed decline. In addition, in the six states consistently monitored by the Centers for Disease Control Pediatric Nutrition Surveillance System, the overall prevalence of anemia declined from 7.8% in 1975 to 2.9% in 1985 (22). Since a significant decline was observed among children seen at pre-enrollment screening visits at public health clinics, as well as those seen at follow-up visits, a generalized improvement in childhood iron nutritional status is likely. In addition, a study of health records from public health clinics in the state of Tennessee revealed that the prevalence of anemia declined significantly within specific socioeconomic groups (22).

A similar decline in the prevalence of anemia, defined as hematocrit of less than 33%, has been reported in a suburban pediatric office from 1969 to 1986 for patients 9 to 23 months of age. The prevalence of anemia was 7.5% during the period from 1969 to 1973 and fell to 2.8% during the period from 1982 to 1986 (23). Likewise, a similar decline has also been observed among 12-month-old children in the Hadera subdistrict of Israel (24).

Iron deficiency anemia still occurs with a much higher frequency among urban infants who are not enrolled in programs such as WIC that provide iron-fortified formulas during the first year of life. Iron deficiency anemia was observed in 20% and iron deficiency without anemia in 29% of 12-month-old infants living in a British inner city (25). In Montreal, iron deficiency anemia was found in 11.4% of Chinese infants 6 to 12 months of age (26). In Syracuse, New York, the incidence of iron deficiency was found to be significantly greater in black infants (14.3%) than in white infants (2.7%) 9 to 12 months of age, although the incidence of iron deficiency without anemia was the same (19.7%) for both whites and blacks (27). Inner-city infants between 6 and 12 months of age not provided with an iron-fortified formula were found to have a 17.4% incidence of iron deficiency and a 24.6% incidence of iron deficiency anemia when they were tested at 1 year of age. In contrast, infants from the same inner-city background who were provided with an iron-fortified formula during the first year of life had only a 1% incidence of iron deficiency (28).

No studies are available that contrast the effects of socioeconomic status on the prevalence of iron deficiency when the diets of the children were comparable. The high prevalence of iron deficiency among infants from lower socioeconomic backgrounds may be a reflection of inadequate dietary iron intake, possibly coupled with an increased infection rate, rather than any mysterious effect of class alone. In studies in which the iron intake was adequate, the prevalence of iron deficiency and iron deficiency anemia in both high- and low-socioeconomic-group infants was apparently the same.

ROLE OF BLOOD LOSS IN THE GENESIS OF IRON DEFICIENCY

The consumption of whole cow's milk during the first year of life repeatedly has been linked to iron deficiency anemia. Hunter, in one of the early prospective studies of infants receiving "private pediatric care," reported that infants fed whole cow's milk from early infancy had a 59% incidence of iron deficiency anemia and a 33% incidence of iron deficiency without anemia (29). More recently, it has been reported that among infants who were fed whole milk before 6 months of age, the incidence of iron deficiency was 62.1% at 9 to 12 months of age, as contrasted with an incidence of 6.5% when the introduction of whole milk was delayed beyond 9 to 10.5 months of age (27). Dine, in a survey of his private practice, found that the response to the question, "How much homogenized milk does your child drink in a day?," identified the patients with iron deficiency as accurately as the determination of the ratio of free erythrocyte porphyrin to hematocrit (30). Infants with iron deficiency consumed at least 1 quart of milk/day. In addition, in a study of London infants, the early introduction of whole cow's milk was found to be a significant dietary variable in the genesis of iron deficiency at 1 year of age (25).

The ingestion of whole cow's milk in infancy is linked to iron deficiency not only because it is a poor source of bioavailable iron, but because it can increase the infant's iron requirement by producing occult gastrointestinal blood loss. The presence of occult enteric blood is a common finding among infants with iron deficiency anemia. Approximately one-half of such infants have blood in their stools (31,32), and blood loss may average 1.45 ml/day (32).

Wilson and associates were the first to implicate the ingestion of whole cow's milk as a cause of gastrointestinal bleeding (33). Using radiolabeled red blood cells, they found that 17 of 34 infants with iron deficiency anemia had occult gastrointestinal bleeding that was induced by the consumption of whole milk. The bleeding was reduced or stopped when soy or other heat-treated proprietary formulas were substituted for whole cow's milk.

Anyon and Clarkson, in a prospective study, reported that 44% of infants receiving a diet of whole cow's milk had occult blood in the stool at 4 months of age, and 27% had positive findings on one or more tests at 8 months of age (34). In infants with demonstrated occult bleeding at 4 months of age, 21% had hemoglobin concentrations of less than 9.5 g/dl by 1 year of age.

In a U.S. study, Fomon and associates found that a greater percentage of infants fed whole cow's milk had positive tests for occult blood between 112 and 140 days than infants fed either a commercial infant formula or a heat-treated milk (35). However, after 140 days of age, there was no difference between groups in the number of stools with occult blood.

The mechanism by which whole milk induces bleeding is unknown, however, intestinal sensitivity to a protein component of milk, such as lactoalbumin, which can be modified by heat processing, may be responsible (36). The proclivity of whole milk to induce bleeding is believed to become less frequent during the second half of the first year of life, although this sensitivity may persist into the second year in selected patients.

SUMMARY

Iron deficiency in infancy is gradually declining in prevalence, probably as a consequence of alterations in infant feeding practices. The increase in the incidence of human milk feeding, the increase in the use of iron-fortified formulas, and the delayed introduction of whole cow's milk all appear to be responsible for the gradual eradication of this preventable nutritional deficiency.

REFERENCES

1. Iob, V., and Swanson, W. W. (1924): Mineral growth of the human fetus. *Am. J. Dis. Child.*, 41:688.
2. Widdowson, E. M., and Spray, C. M. (1951): Chemical development in utero. *Arch. Dis. Child.*, 26:205.
3. Osgood, E. E. (1955): Development and growth of hematopoietic tissues. *Pediatrics*, 15:733.
4. Pribilla, W., Bothwell, T., and Finch, C. A. (1958): Iron transport to the fetus in man. In: *Iron in Clinical Medicine*, edited by R. O. Wallerstein and S. R. Mettier. University of California Press, Los Angeles, p. 58.
5. Loh, T. T., Higuchi, D. A., Van Bockxmeer, F. M., et al. (1980): Transferrin receptors on the human placental microvillus membrane. *J. Clin. Invest.*, 65:1182.
6. Woodruff, C. W., and Bridgeforth, E. B. (1953): Relationship between the hemogram of the infant and that of the mother during pregnancy. *Pediatrics*, 12:681.
7. Lanzkowsky, P. (1961): The influence of maternal iron deficiency on the hemoglobin of the infant. *Arch. Dis. Child.*, 36:205.
8. Ogunbode, O. (1980): The relationship between hematocrit levels in gravidae and their newborn. *Int. J. Gynaecol. Obstet.*, 18:57.
9. Sisson, T. R. C., and Lund, C. J. (1957): The influence of maternal iron deficiency on the newborn. *Am. J. Dis. Child.*, 94:525.
10. Singla, P. N., Chand, S., Khanna, S., et al. (1978): Effect of maternal anemia on the placenta and newborn infant. *Acta Paediatr. Scand.*, 67:645.
11. Zittoun, J., Blot, I., Hill, C., et al. (1983): Iron supplements versus placebo during pregnancy: its effects on iron and folate status of mothers and newborns. *Ann. Nutr. Metab.*, 27:320.
12. Rios, E., Lipschitz, D. A., Cook, J. D., et al. (1975): Relationship of maternal and infant iron stores as assessed by determination of plasma ferritin. *Pediatrics*, 55:694.
13. Nemet, K., Andrassy, K., Bornar, K., et al. (1986): Relationship between maternal and infant iron stores. 1. Full term infants. *Haematolgia*, 19:197.
14. Chong, S. K. F., Thompson, J. E. H., and Barltrop, D. (1984): Free erythrocyte protoporphyrin as an index of perinatal iron status. *J. Pediatr. Gastroenterol. Nutr.*, 3:224.
15. Oski, F. A. (1980): Anemia in infancy: iron deficiency and vitamin E deficiency. *Pediatr. Rev.*, 1:247.
16. Committee on Nutrition (1969): Iron balance and requirements in infancy. *Pediatrics*, 43:134.
17. Lane, M., and Johnson, C. L. (1981): Prevalence of iron deficiency. In: *Iron Nutrition Revisited—Infancy, Childhood, Adolescence. Report of the 82nd Ross Conference on Pediatric Research*, edited by F. A. Oski and H. A. Pearson. Ross Laboratories, Columbus, OH, pp. 31–46.

18. Johnson, C. L., and Abraham, S. (1979): Hemoglobin and selected iron-related findings of persons 1–74 years of age: United States, 1971–74. Advanced data from Vital and Health Statistics, No. 46, National Center for Health Statistics.
19. Picciano, M. F., and Deering, R. H. (1980): The influence of feeding regimens on iron status during infancy. *Am. J. Clin. Nutr.*, 33:746.
20. Miller, V., Swaney, S., and Deinard, A. S. (1985): Impact of the WIC program on the iron status of infants. *Pediatrics*, 75:100.
21. Vasquez-Seoane, P., Windom, R., and Pearson, H. A. (1985): Disappearance of iron deficiency anemia in a high risk population given supplemental iron. *N. Engl. J. Med.*, 313:1239–1240.
22. Yip, R., Binkin, N. J., Fleshood, L., et al. (1987): Declining prevalence of anemia among low-income children in the United States. *JAMA*, 257:1619.
23. Yip, R., Walsh, K. M., Goldfarb, M., et al. (1987): Declining childhood anemia prevalence in a middle-class setting: a pediatric success story. *Pediatrics*, 80:330.
24. Rishpon, S. (1986): Prevalence rate of anemia among 12-month-old children in the Hadera sub-district, Israel, 1984–85. *Israel J. Med. Sci.*, 22:412.
25. Morton, R. E., Nysenbaum, A., and Price, K. (1988): Iron status in the first year of life. *J. Pediatr. Gastroenterol. Nutr.*, 7:707.
26. Chan-Yip, A., and Gray-Donald, K. (1987): Prevalence of iron deficiency among Chinese children aged 6 to 36 months in Montreal. *Can. Med. Assoc. J.*, 136:373.
27. Sadowitz, P. D., and Oski, F. A. (1983): Iron status and infant feeding practices in an urban ambulatory center. *Pediatrics*, 72:33.
28. Tunnessen, W. W., and Oski, F. A. (1987): Consequences of starting whole cow milk at 6 months of age. *J. Pediatr.*, 111:813.
29. Hunter, R. (1970): Iron nutrition in infancy. In: *Report of the 62nd Ross Conference on Pediatric Research*. Ross Laboratories, Columbus, OH, p. 22.
30. Dine, M. S. (1980): Evaluation of the free erythrocyte porphyrin (FEP) test in a private practice. The incidence of iron deficiency and increased lead absorption in 9- to 13-month-old-infants. *Pediatrics*, 65:303.
31. Morton, R. E., Njysenbaum, A., and Price, K. (1988): Iron status in the first year of life. *J. Pediatr. Gastroenterol. Nutr.*, 7:707.
32. Rasch, C. A., Cotton, E. K., Harris, J. W., et al. (1960): Blood loss as a contributing factor in the etiology of iron-lack anemia in infancy. *Am. J. Dis. Child.*, 100:627.
33. Hoag, M. S., Wallerstein, R. O., and Pollycove, M. (1961): Occult blood loss in iron deficiency anemia of infancy. *Pediatrics*, 27:199.
34. Wilson, J. F., Lahey, M. E., and Heiner, D. C. (1974): Studies on iron metabolism. V. Further observations on cow's milk-induced gastrointestinal bleeding in infants with iron-deficiency anemia. *J. Pediatr.*, 84:335.
35. Anyon, C. P., and Clarkson, K. G. (1971): Cows' milk: a cause of iron deficiency anemia in infants. *N.Z. Med. J.*, 74:24.
36. Fomon, S. J., Ziegler, E. E., Nelson, S. E., et al. (1981): Cow milk feeding in infancy: gastrointestinal blood loss and iron nutritional status. *J. Pediatr.*, 98:540.
37. Dallman, P. R., Siimes, M. A., and Stekel, A. (1980): Iron deficiency in infancy and childhood. *Am. J. Clin. Nutr.*, 33:86.

Dietary Iron: Birth to Two Years,
edited by L. J. Filer, Jr.
Raven Press, Ltd., New York © 1989.

Discussion

Dr. Walter: Would you comment on the 11.7% anemia rate in the iron-fortified formula group at 12 months?

Dr. Oski: That was the percentage who had hemoglobin values of less than 11 g/dl. Some of these children did not meet other criteria for iron deficiency anemia. However, if one analyzes all of the data for the infants with hemoglobin levels that are less than 11 g/dl and subjects them to multiple iron deficiency analysis, such as the type that Dr. Yip referred to, the incidence is about 2%.

Dr. Walter: What was the mean hemoglobin value?

Dr. Oski: The hemoglobin levels were slightly and statistically significantly higher in the iron-fortified formula group. I broke the data down this way to illustrate more dramatically the tendency for the distribution curve to shift to the left in this group of infants.

Dr. Owen: What was the racial makeup of the study comparing infants who received iron-fortified formula to those receiving cow milk.

Dr. Oski: The racial makeup in that particular study was approximately 50% black and 50% white.

Dr. Walter: I would like to add to the information presented by Dr. Oski on gastrointestinal bleeding in infants. In a study of 40 infants, including a group under 4 months of age and a group 7 to 9 months of age, we fed four different formulas for 10 days each. These formulas were powdered whole cow's milk, unmodified homogenized cow's milk, a milk-based infant formula, and a soy isolate formula. The formulas were used sequentially, but the sequence of treatments was different in the different groups. The numbers of infants receiving each milk were not equal because some of the infants exited the study before completing the feeding sequence. We gave the infants the feedings for 7 days and collected their diapers between two labels of crystal blue on the last 3 days. We measured the hemoglobin content of the stools using a fluorescent test for hemoglobin called Hemoquant. Mean blood loss of the infants fed powdered milk was 0.07 ml of blood/day (identical to the normal values reported by Wilson), 0.09 ml when fed fresh milk, 0.04 ml when fed the milk-based formula, and 0.05 ml when fed the soy isolate–based formula. The order of treatment did not influence the results. The differences were very highly significant according to a one-way analysis of variance. Fresh cow's milk, in infants up to 9 months of age, induces greater blood loss than any of the heat-treated milk formulas or soy-based formulas.

Dr. Oski: It appears that some of those infants had a fairly high blood loss to produce such a large standard deviation.

Dr. Walter: That is correct.

Dr. Yip: Based on your sample size, any difference in the mean value of more than 0.01 ml will be found to be statistically significant according to the test of means.

Dr. Ziegler: Is the powdered milk more heat-treated than pasteurized milk?

Dr. Walter: Yes. It is heated to 160 or 180°F.

Dr. Ziegler: Is it less heat-treated than the milk-based formula?

Dr. Walter: It is heat-treated about the same.

Dr. Filer: I used to think that powdered formula received more heat treatment than liquid formula, but I have been told that this is not so and that powdered formulas actually receive significantly less heat treatment than liquid formulas.

Dr. Walter: The old studies use fresh homogenized milk that was apparently not treated with a deodorization stage that the F.I.L. requires. In this procedure the milk is heated to about 80° for several seconds at the end of the procedure. This has been done now for the past decade or so. We thought this might be enough to eliminate the difference between homogenized milk and heat-treated milks, but evidently it does not.

Dr. Filer: Dr. Oski, would you comment on other nutritional factors, such as phytates, tannins, and ascorbic acid, and their role in iron deficiency?

Dr. Oski: Dr. Dallman mentioned the study, from Israel, of children fed tea early in life who develop iron deficiency. There are studies from developing countries suggesting that vitamin A deficiency mimics iron deficiency in many of its laboratory manifestations. We probably should examine the vitamin A status of some of the children who are labeled iron-deficient in the U.S. recognizing that vitamin A deficiency is probably very unlikely.

Dr. Filer: Is the vitamin A affecting the gut epithelium?

Dr. Oski: The mechanism has not been worked out but it clearly produces a hypochromic microcytic anemia that is not responsive to iron therapy.

Dr. Walravens: Suppose you have a child who is presumably iron-deficient; you give him iron and nothing happens. You give him some vitamin drops and the anemia is cured within a month with an increase of 1 g/dl in hemoglobin or a change in whatever criteria you use. Do you think that this is related to a possible vitamin A deficiency?

Dr. Oski: I have to say that I have never given extra vitamins and observed that. I have always assumed that there was no reason to be looking for anything else. Have you seen cases like that?

Dr. Walravens: Occasionally.

Dr. Oski: It might have been a child who had some recent fat malabsorption and became vitamin A–deficient and it may have appeared to be an iron deficiency but the child did not respond to iron.

Dr. Walravens: Could you comment on iron-deficient patients who do not absorb iron?

Dr. Oski: There are some reports that a very small percentage of children who are iron-deficient have iron malabsorption. We did a prospective study to determine the incidence of iron malabsorption and found that about 4% of all iron-deficient and anemic children had flat iron absorption curves and we gave them parenteral iron to normalize their absorption. There was a study from South America by Dr. George Graham that identified a much higher incidence of iron malabsorption, but he was studying iron deficiency anemia and not just mild iron deficiency. We know that iron deficiency usually results in increased iron absorption; however, when patients become very iron-deficient, the percent of iron absorption decreases. A number of years ago, Weintraub bled a group of puppies making them progressively more and more iron-deficient and anemic during the first 6 months of life. While they were becoming profoundly iron deficient and anemic, their iron absorption increased. When their hematocrits were about 15%, iron absorption decreased. He treated these puppies with intramuscular iron and their ability to absorb iron increased within days. There are some suggestive studies to indicate that with profound iron deficiency anemia, there are mucosal alterations in the gut that might be responsible for these observations.

Dr. Ziegler: In those human studies that associated iron deficiency with mucosal alterations, they not only treated them with iron but also put them on a milk-free, gluten-free diet. Isn't that correct?

Dr. Oski: I was one of the authors of that study. We did not eliminate the possibility that the alterations were induced by whole cow's milk and were not the results of iron deficiency alone. These were often children who had been drinking 1 to 2 quarts of cow's milk per day. They had occult gastrointestinal bleeding and we gave them parenteral iron. Their iron losses were not altered until they were taken off milk. Studies by Calvin Woodruff showed the same results.

Dr. Dallman: You mentioned some of the early studies on intestinal blood losses in which the children had fairly severe anemias. I was thinking about the study by Marty Siimes of children with gluten enteropathy who continued to have blood loss even after their diet was corrected. Are there actually two types of problems? There is the situation in which there are milk-related blood losses that happen in a very large percentage of children. That is not really an idiosyncrasy. Rather, it is almost like aspirin-induced blood losses that occur in almost everybody. In contrast, there are the almost idiosyncratic reactions of gluten enteropathy and protein-losing enteropathy that are relatively rare and the literature sometimes confuses these two situations.

Dr. Oski: There are some studies in which cow's milk was given and within 48 hr there were mucosal alterations demonstrated by jejunal biopsies. I really do not know how common the problem is.

Dietary Iron: Birth to Two Years,
edited by L. J. Filer, Jr.
Raven Press, Ltd., New York © 1989.

Intestinal Blood Loss by Normal Infants Fed Cow's Milk

Ekhard E. Ziegler

Department of Pediatrics, College of Medicine, University of Iowa, Iowa City, Iowa 52242

In the 1960s, it was recognized that intestinal blood loss could cause iron deficiency anemia (1,2). Furthermore, Wilson et al. (3), using ^{51}Cr-tagged erythrocytes, furnished convincing evidence that intestinal blood loss could be provoked by the feeding of cow's milk. These investigators also showed that the effect of cow's milk was dose-dependent and could be abolished by heat treatment of cow's milk (of a more extensive kind than mere pasteurization). The studies of Elian et al. (4), also using ^{51}Cr-tagged erythrocytes, showed that virtually all otherwise normal infants lose small amounts of blood with their stool. However, the number of infants in this study (4) was small, and it remained unclear whether intestinal blood loss was a universal phenomenon. Also, it has remained unclear whether cow's milk could induce intestinal blood loss in normal (nonanemic) infants and, if so, whether blood loss by normal infants could be of sufficient magnitude to affect iron nutritional status.

Initial information on this question was provided by Woodruff et al. (5) from a prospective study of normal infants. The infants were breast-fed or formula-fed up to 2 months of age and then fed whole cow's milk (13 infants) or a non-iron-fortified formula (25 infants). A sensitive guaiac test was used to detect the presence of blood in the stools, and a number of positive reactions were detected even in feces of fully breast-fed infants. Among formula-fed infants at 3, 6, 9, and 12 months of age, guaiac-positive stools were detected in 44, 52, 67, and 54% of stools, respectively. Among infants fed cow's milk, the corresponding percentages were 92, 69, 83, and 64% at 3, 6, 9, and 12 months of age, respectively. Thus, a greater percentage of guaiac-positive stools was seen in infants fed whole cow's milk than in infants fed formula, although it was not possible to judge the nutritional significance of the blood loss in either group. The study failed to provide evidence that younger infants were more susceptible than older infants to cow's milk-provoked gastrointestinal blood loss.

In this study by Woodruff et al. (5), intakes of iron were similar for the infants fed the non-iron-fortified formula and those fed cow's milk. Blood samples were obtained at 3, 6, 9, and 12 months of age. In the group fed whole cow's milk, hemoglobin concentration was significantly less at ages 9 and 12 months, and mean corpuscular volume and percent saturation of transferrin were significantly less at 6 and 9 months of age. Thus, this study provided some evidence that the feeding of cow's milk had adverse effects on iron nutritional status over a long period.

In a study somewhat similar in design to that of Woodruff et al., except that the observation periods were shorter, Fomon et al. (6) observed 81 normal infants from 112 to 196 days of age who were divided into three feeding groups. One group was fed a low-iron, milk-based formula, one group was fed homogenized whole cow's milk heat-treated in the same manner as the infant formula, and one group was fed pasteurized, homogenized whole cow's milk. All infants received a daily supplement providing 12 mg of iron as ferrous sulfate. In most instances, a stool sample was collected each week and tested with the guaiac reaction. Figure 1 indicates the percent guaiac-positive stools in each group at baseline (112 days of age), from 119 to 140 days of age, from 147 to 168 days of age, and from 175 to 196 days of age. The number of infants with guaiac-positive stools and the total number of guaiac-positive stools during the first 28 days of the trial (from 119 to 140 days of age) was significantly greater in the group fed whole cow's milk than in the other groups ($p < 0.01$ and < 0.001, respectively). During the later

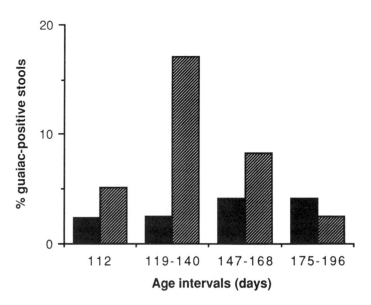

FIG. 1. Percent of stools with positive guaiac reaction (■) of infants fed formula or heat-treated cow's milk and (▨) of infants fed cow's milk after 112 days of age. (Reproduced from ref. 6 with permission, © C.V. Mosby Co., 1981.)

periods, differences in percent of subjects with guaiac-positive stools and in total number of guaiac-positive stools in the three feeding groups were small and not statistically significant. As was the case with the study reported by Woodruff et al. (5), the clinical significance of these observations was difficult to evaluate because guaiac tests do not yield quantitative data on blood loss. No differences were detected in iron nutritional status between the various feeding groups. However, iron intakes were generous, and the observation period was short.

With the availability in recent years of quantitative tests of fecal hemoglobin, it has become possible to determine the extent of fecal blood loss. In a recently completed study of normal infants fed either cow's milk or a milk-based formula (Ziegler et al., to be published), we have used a sensitive and specific method (7) for the quantitative determination of fecal loss of hemoglobin. With this method, it is possible to detect 0.02 mg of hemoglobin/g of wet feces. From 168 through 252 days of age, 26 infants were fed cow's milk, and 26 infants were fed a low-iron, milk-based formula. Selected other foods low in iron content were permitted, and one jar per day of a specially prepared cereal–fruit combination providing 3.65 mg of iron in the form of ferrous sulfate was provided. Before entering the trial, all infants had been fed a milk-based formula with 12 mg of iron per liter for 28 days or more. Thirty-one infants had been breast-fed, whereas 21 infants had never been breast-fed. Stool samples were collected before the start of the trial (at 140, 166, 167, and 168 days of age) and at weekly intervals thereafter for determination of hemoglobin concentration. In addition, stools were tested for occult blood with the guaiac reaction (Hemoccult, Smith Kline Diagnostics, Sunnyvale, CA, U.S.A.). Venous blood was obtained in most cases at 140 days of age and during the trial at 168, 196, 224, and 252 days of age for determination of hematocrit, hemoglobin concentration, erythrocyte protoporphyrin, serum iron, and ferritin.

As shown in Fig. 2, the percent of guaiac-positive stools was significantly greater ($p < 0.01$) in the group fed cow's milk than in the group fed formula during the first 28 days of the trial (175 to 196 days of age). Differences in the percent of guaiac-positive stools were smaller and not statistically significant during the two subsequent 28-day periods. Results of quantitive determinations of fecal hemoglobin indicated that the group fed cow's milk had much higher fecal hemoglobin losses than the group fed formula (Fig. 3). The difference was statistically significant in each 28-day period. Closer inspection of the data revealed that six infants fed cow's milk showed no appreciable increase above baseline in fecal hemoglobin loss ("nonresponders"). Responses of the other 20 ("responders") infants were highly variable, and most infants had increased hemoglobin loss even in the first stool sample obtained after starting on cow's milk (at 175 days of age). In many infants, fecal hemoglobin loss declined later, but a few infants had sustained high hemoglobin losses. In some infants, fecal hemoglobin loss did not

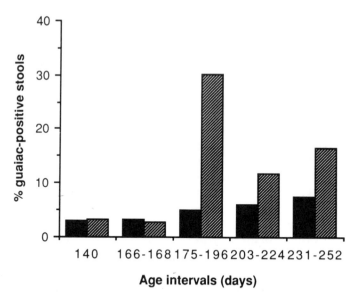

FIG. 2. Percent of stools with positive guaiac reaction (■) of infants fed formula and (▨) of infants fed cow's milk after 168 days of age.

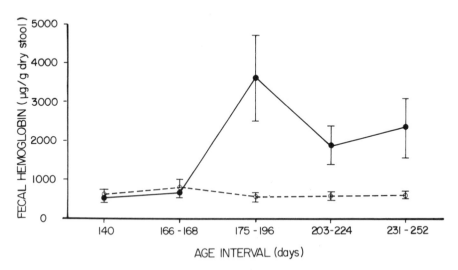

FIG. 3. Fecal hemoglobin concentration of infants (○) fed formula and infants (●) fed cow's milk after 168 days of age. Bars indicate standard error.

TABLE 1. *Indices of iron nutritional status*

	\multicolumn{10}{c}{Age (days)}									
	140		168		196		224		252	
	Mean	SD	Mean	SD	Mean	SD	Mean	SD	Mean	SD
Hemoglobin (g/dl)										
Cow's milk	11.8	1.1	11.8	0.9	11.7	0.9	11.8	1.0	12.0	0.9
Formula	11.9	1.0	12.1	1.1	11.8	1.0	11.9	1.0	12.1	0.6
Hematocrit (%)										
Cow's milk	35.2	2.6	35.4	2.9	35.9	2.2	36.1	2.5	36.4	2.7
Formula	35.3	2.1	35.4	1.7	35.4	2.0	35.6	1.8	36.2	1.7
Serum iron (µg/dl)										
Cow's milk	46.1	17.8	55.8	21.4	47.9	16.7	41.1	14.5	49.5	25.1
Formula	45.2	14.6	55.5	18.5	48.9	13.8	48.5	20.3	52.3	25.1
Ferritin (ng/ml)										
Cow's milk	64.9	51.0	36.4	34.8	33.7	32.1	20.9	11.9	25.1	13.6
Formula	64.3	48.0	52.8	31.4	42.4	39.2	28.0	19.7	19.6	11.7
EP (µg/dl)										
Cow's milk	59.7	22.0	49.4	19.9	77.6	53.2	64.7	25.4	70.8	19.0
Formula	89.2	31.4	63.2	20.5	67.4	15.0	58.9	15.4	60.2	17.0

EP, erythrocyte protoporphyrin.

increase until several weeks after cow's milk feeding was started. Mean fecal hemoglobin of the 20 responders was 4,773 µg/g of dry stool during the period 175 to 196 days of age.

Assuming a wet stool weight of 60 g/day with 20% dry solids, a fecal hemoglobin concentration of 4,773 µg/g of dry stool represents an iron loss of 0.20 mg/day, a quantity we consider nutritionally significant.

Biochemical indices of iron nutritional status did not differ between the group fed cow's milk and the group fed formula. As shown in Table 1, hematocrit and concentrations of hemoglobin, erythrocyte protoporphyrin, serum iron, and ferritin provided no evidence for deterioration of iron nutritional status among infants fed cow's milk. There was also no difference in iron nutritional status between responders and nonresponders in the group fed cow's milk. However, one infant with high fecal blood loss developed clear evidence of iron deficiency within 4 weeks after cow's milk was introduced.

CONCLUSIONS

The literature and our own studies provide convincing evidence that consumption of cow's milk leads to increased gastrointestinal blood loss in the majority of normal, nonanemic infants. The data do not suggest that susceptibility to cow's milk-induced blood loss is age-dependent during the first year of life. However, blood loss is most severe when cow's milk is first introduced and diminishes in most infants with the duration of feeding cow's milk. A few infants experience quite large blood loss, but the data are insufficient to estimate the prevalence of this phenomenon.

In our studies, few adverse effects on iron nutritional status have been evident, presumably because of the relatively short exposure to cow's milk (3 months). Studies with longer periods of cow's milk feeding have generally demonstrated impaired iron nutritional status. Thus, there can be little question that the feeding of cow's milk to infants and young children for a prolonged period is likely to lead to poor iron nutritional status and, in some infants, to outright iron deficiency. The relative importance of gastrointestinal blood loss, displacement by cow's milk of more iron-rich foods, and inhibition of iron absorption remains to be determined. We conclude that cow's milk is an unsuitable food during the first year of life.

REFERENCES

1. Rasch, C. A., Cotton, E. K., Harris, J. W., and Griggs, R. C. (1960): Blood loss as a contributing factor in the etiology of iron-lack anemia of infancy. *Am. J. Dis. Child.*, 100:627(Abstract).
2. Hoag, M. S., Wallerstein, R. O., and Pollycove, M. (1961): Occult blood loss in iron deficiency anemia of infancy. *Pediatrics*, 27:199–203.
3. Wilson, J. F., Lahey, M. E., and Heiner, D. C. (1974): Studies on iron metabolism. *J. Pediatr.*, 84:335–344.
4. Elian, E., Bar-Shani, S., Liberman, A., and Matoth, Y. (1966): Intestinal blood loss: a factor in calculations of body iron in late infancy. *J. Pediatr.*, 69:215–219.
5. Woodruff, C. W., Wright, S. W., and Wright, R. P. (1972): The role of fresh cow's milk in iron deficiency. *Am. J. Dis. Child.*, 124:26–30.
6. Fomon, S. J., Ziegler, E. E., Nelson, S. E., and Edwards, B. B. (1981): Cow milk feeding in infancy: gastrointestinal blood loss and iron nutritional status. *J. Pediatr.*, 98:540–545.
7. Schwartz, S., Dahl, J., Ellefson, M., and Ahlquist, D. (1983): The HemoQuant test: a specific and quantitative determination of heme (hemoglobin) in feces and other materials. *Clin. Chem.*, 29:2061–2067.

Dietary Iron: Birth to Two Years,
edited by L. J. Filer, Jr.
Raven Press, Ltd., New York © 1989.

Discussion

Dr. Filer: In the study comparing cow's milk with heat-treated cow milk, was the ascorbic acid intake controlled?

Dr. Ziegler: Ascorbic acid was not given to the infants fed cow's milk; however, the formula contained at least 50 mg/liter; thus, infants fed formula received more vitamin C.

Dr. Walravens: Which fruits did you use in the iron-fortified cereal–fruit combination?

Dr. Ziegler: Bananas and pears. These products were fortified with vitamin C.

Dr. Walter: Did the infants receive meat?

Dr. Ziegler: No.

Dr. Dallman: In your second study in which you changed the feedings of formula-fed and breast-fed infants to cow's milk, how many were breast-fed?

Dr. Ziegler: Thirty-one were breast-fed, and the other 21 were formula-fed.

Dr. Walravens: What was the weight of the dry stool in this study?

Dr. Ziegler: We assumed that it was 10 to 12 g. Stool dry solids account for around 23% to 25% of stool weight.

Dr. Filer: Was there any relationship between iron loss and the use of solid foods?

Dr. Ziegler: No. Solid foods were started at 140 days and were limited to one jar of the fruit–cereal mixture.

Dr. Filer: So, you never eliminated solid foods.

Dr. Ziegler: In this study, we did not.

Dr. Walter: Was the infant who had the high iron loss breast-fed in early life?

Dr. Ziegler: Yes, she was, but only for about 1 month.

Dr. Walter: In our study, infants who were fed fresh cow's milk had almost double the stool volume than infants receiving either milk or soy formula and somewhat more stool volume than when they were fed powdered milk.

Dr. Ziegler: That parallels our observations. Infants fed cow's milk had lower dry solid concentrations in their stools than infants who were fed formulas.

Dr. Walter: In our longitudinal studies, about one-third of infants, despite having the same birth weight and living in the same environment and receiving the same diet, develop iron deficiency anemia. Another one-third have biochemical evidence of iron deficiency and another one-third have normal iron status. Our question has always been: why is there a difference in large groups of infants who are essentially the same? Our current longitudinal study is a follow-up of a large number of infants to find out if there is a group of infants who have increased iron loss and, as a result, eventually become anemic. These infants are receiving modified formula and powdered milk. None of the infants are receiving fresh cow's milk, which is normally not consumed by infants in Chile. From our daily stool collections, we have found that a few of the infants tend to lose more blood, as indicated by Dr. Ziegler.

Dr. Dallman: Did you obtain a family history of allergy?

Dr. Ziegler: No, we did not obtain such histories. We recently inquired about the infant who had high stool blood losses to determine how she was doing. She is a perfectly normal child without any signs of gastrointestinal illness.

Dr. Oski: Did she have atopic dermatitis? Sometimes, cow's milk protein causes both gastrointestinal symptoms and atopic dermatitis.

Dr. Ziegler: There was no clinical evidence of atopic dermatitis.

Dr. Filer: Allergic infants may also have colitis. At what age are stool blood losses an issue? It is frequently recommended that cow's milk not be introduced before 1 year of age, but is 1 year too early?

Dr. Ziegler: Our study went only to age 252 days. Wilson et al. (1974) observed that some infants have blood loss into the second year of life. But, in addition, they showed that infants who have this problem in infancy have no blood loss when they ingest cow's milk later in life. Formerly, my primary reason for recommending against cow's milk feeding during infancy was renal solute load. Now, I feel the main concern is blood loss.

Dietary Iron: Birth to Two Years,
edited by L.J. Filer, Jr.
Raven Press, Ltd., New York © 1989.

Bioavailability of Iron from Infant Foods: Studies with Stable Isotopes

Ekhard E. Ziegler

Department of Pediatrics, College of Medicine, University of Iowa, Iowa City, Iowa 52242

Iron deficiency is common among infants and young children both in industrialized and in developing countries (1). Besides inadequate intake of iron, poor availability of ingested iron is a major cause of poor iron nutriture. Development of strategies to combat iron deficiency has been impeded by lack of precise information about the availability to infants and young children of food iron and fortification iron. This lack of information is due to a reluctance to use radioisotopes in studies of infants and young children, although administration of radioiron poses a very negligible hazard. However, the use of stable (nonradioactive) isotopes has recently become feasible as a result of the development of suitable mass spectrometry instrumentation, such as inductively coupled plasma mass spectrometry (ICP/MS). The feasibility of using ^{58}Fe, the least abundant stable isotope of iron (natural abundance 0.322 weight%), for studies of iron metabolism in infants has been demonstrated (2,3). Enrichment of circulating erythrocyte iron following administration of a tracer amount of ^{58}Fe can be determined with sufficient precision to permit use of the erythrocyte incorporation approach for comparative studies. This approach is more convenient than the isotope balance method, which requires prolonged periods of stool collection.

GENERAL METHODOLOGY OF STABLE ISOTOPE STUDIES OF IRON

Whole body counting following the administration of radioiron (^{55}Fe or ^{59}Fe) is considered the most precise method to determine iron bioavailability (4). Obviously, an equivalent approach does not exist for stable isotopes. Since the cumbersome nature of isotope balance studies limits their use, erythrocyte incorporation studies are the approach of choice for availability studies with the use of stable isotopes. The main limitation of this approach is that the percentage of absorbed iron that is promptly incorporated into hemoglobin and that appears in circulating erythrocytes is unknown. In normal and in iron-deficient adults, that percentage is greater than 80% and usually around 90% (1), so that, to estimate actual absorption, an arbitrary correction must be made. However, this limitation is not an impediment in studies of the relative bioavailability of iron, where it is sufficient to state results in terms of the percentage of administered label found in circulating erythrocytes. Naturally, the conditions of administration and measurement must be rigorously standardized.

Two additional points concerning stable isotope studies must be mentioned. First, a background correction must always be made since the isotope used as a label is always naturally present, or it may even be present at higher than natural abundance in subjects who have served in earlier similar studies. Second, mass spectrometric measurements of iron yield isotope ratios. Therefore, to calculate the amount of the isotope of interest, the total amount of the element must be determined independently. In the case of erythrocyte incorporation studies of iron, the total amount of circulating iron is estimated from the determined blood hemoglobin concentration and an assumed blood volume.

Finally, in studies of iron bioavailability, wide interindividual variability of values is universally observed, even among subjects with proven good iron nutritional status. It is therefore customary in studies with radioisotopes of iron to administer a second isotope as a reference dose (e.g., as ferrous ascorbate) in close temporal proximity to the test dose, and to correct results with the first isotope for the value obtained with the reference isotope. In the case of stable isotopes, this approach is not yet possible.

FEASIBILITY OF STABLE ISOTOPE STUDIES IN INFANTS

In a feasibility study (3), nine normal healthy infants were studied at 126 days of age. Between 8 and 112 days of age, these infants had served as subjects in studies of food intake and growth and had received various formulas providing at least 1.8 mg of iron/100 kcal. From 112 to 128 days of age, a milk-based formula providing about 0.2 mg of iron/100 kcal was fed. At 126 days of age, the infants received the test dose of ^{58}Fe. The dose consisted of 1.95 mg of iron containing 1.44 mg of ^{58}Fe as ferrous sulfate and was administered as a solution containing 84 mg of ascorbic acid and 400 mg of sucrose in a volume of 5 ml. The dose was given 2 hr after a formula feeding and 2 hr before the next feeding. Venous blood was obtained at 84, 112, 140, 168, and 196 days of age for determination of hemoglobin concentration, serum ferritin concentration, and the ^{58}Fe/^{57}Fe mass isotope ratio ($MIR_{58/57}$), the latter by ICP/MS. The coefficient of variation for the isotope ratio determinations was 1% or less. The amount of ^{58}Fe label incorporated into erythrocytes ($^{58}Fe_{inc}$) at time t after the administration of ^{58}Fe label was calculated as follows:

$$^{58}Fe_{inc} = \frac{MIR^t_{58/57} - MIR^0_{58/57}}{MIR^0_{58/57}} \times Fe_{circ} \times 0.00322$$

where $^{58}Fe_{inc}$ is expressed in mg, $MIR^t_{58/57}$ is the determined $MIR_{58/57}$ at time t after dosing, $MIR^0_{58/57}$ is the baseline ratio, Fe_{circ} is the amount of total circulating iron (mg) at time t, and 0.00322 is the natural abundance (weight fraction) of ^{58}Fe. This calculation corrects for the natural abundance of ^{58}Fe. Thus, $^{58}Fe_{inc}$ represents label ^{58}Fe that appears in erythrocytes at time t. It is usually expressed as a percentage of the label dose. The amount of total circulating iron (mg) was estimated as $Fe_{circ} = BV \times Hgb \times 3.47$, where BV is the blood volume in ml, assumed to be 65 ml/kg of body weight, Hgb is the hemoglobin concentration in g/ml, and 3.47 is the concentration of iron in hemoglobin (mg/g).

Individual values for the $^{58}Fe/^{57}Fe$ ratio in circulating erythrocytes are presented in Fig. 1. It is evident that the ratio is elevated (i.e., enrichment of erythrocyte iron is increased) 2 weeks after administration of the ^{58}Fe label. The two subjects with the highest enrichment received a second dose

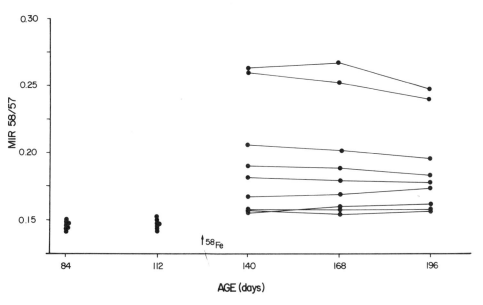

FIG. 1. $MIR_{58/57}$ in circulating erythrocytes before (84 and 112 days of age) and after (140, 168, and 196 days of age) administration of the ^{58}Fe label. (Drawn from data from ref. 3.)

of the [58]Fe label 1 day after the first dose. It is also evident that enrichment is highest at 140 days of age and declines gradually thereafter. The decline is due to expansion of the circulating hemoglobin mass through addition of unlabeled erythrocytes, as evidenced by the fact that the calculated amount of circulating [58]Fe label did not change significantly: the average circulating [58]Fe label was 0.1852 mg at 140 days of age, 0.1882 mg at 168 days of age, and 0.1868 mg at 196 days of age. The data offered the opportunity to obtain an estimate of the overall methodological error, i.e., the error due to uncertainties in the measurement of isotope ratios and of hemoglobin concentrations, as well as uncertainties in the assumed blood volume. Table 1 presents for each subject the mean value (from determinations at 140, 168, and 196 days of age) for circulating [58]Fe label, expressed both in absolute terms (mg) and as percent of the dose. The standard deviation represents an estimate of the uncertainty of the method. Expressed as percent of the dose, the standard deviations ranged from 0.11% to 1.28%. However, expressed as the coefficient of variation, uncertainties ranged from 1.0% to 30.5% of the dose, with a mean of 9.7%. For the six subjects with incorporation greater than 4% of the dose, the mean coefficient of variation was only 5.6%.

The wide interindividual variation of percent incorporation represents a formidable obstacle to comparative studies of iron bioavailability that will be overcome only when a second stable isotope becomes available as a reference dose. Interindividual variation is partly explained by variation in iron nutritional status, which, in turn, is reflected by serum ferritin concentration. Percent [58]Fe label incorporated was inversely correlated with mean ferritin concentration ($r = -0.836$, Spearman rank correlation, $p < 0.01$).

TABLE 1. *Circulating [58]Fe label[a]*

Subject	Mean dose (mg)	Percent of dose		
		Mean	SD	CV
3165	0.4573	15.9	0.62	3.9
3342	0.4613	16.0	0.79	4.9
3166	0.1497	10.4	0.11	1.0
3343	0.1064	7.4	1.28	17.3
3378	0.0537	3.7	1.14	30.5
3379	0.0456	3.2	0.55	17.3
3382	0.0547	3.8	0.23	6.0
3384	0.1385	9.6	0.22	2.2
3391	0.2138	14.8	0.62	4.2
Mean	0.1868	7.9[b]	0.62[c]	9.7[c]

SD = standard deviation; CV = coefficient of variation.
[a]From ref. 3.
[b]Geometric mean.
[c]Arithmetic mean.

IRON ABSORPTION FROM INFANT FOODS

The bioavailability of iron from different infant foods and from different iron salts was assessed in a series of studies (5) using an approach generally similar to that previously described, except that test meals labeled with [58]Fe were fed at 154 days of age. From 112 days of age until 4 days after the day on which the test meal was fed, a milk-based formula providing approximately 0.3 mg of iron/100 kcal was fed. From 140 days of age until 4 days after the test meal, a food similar or identical to that scheduled for use as the test meal was fed at least once daily. Subsequently, infants were permitted to receive other foods. Venous blood was obtained at 140, 168, and 196 days of age. Methods and procedures were as described above. Values for percent erythrocyte incorporation of [58]Fe were calculated separately for each infant at 168 and 196 days of age, and the average value was used.

The results are summarized in Table 2. Four foods were fortified with ferrous sulfate, and one food was fortified with ferrous fumarate. Despite efforts to achieve similar intakes of iron with all test meals, intakes of iron from test meals differed with the different foods for technical reasons. Values for percent incorporation showed wide variability between individual infants. Differences between foods were not statistically significant. It may be concluded that rice cereal does not exert a substantial inhibitory effect on iron absorption. Grape juice, despite its ascorbic acid concentration of 31 mg/100 ml, was not associated with greater iron incorporation than that observed with other foods. Similarly, the relatively small amount of beef (about 1% of wet weight) of the vegetables and beef preparation apparently did not enhance the availability of iron. Finally, the data suggest that iron was as available from ferrous fumarate as from ferrous sulfate. Ferrous fumarate is a promising iron salt for fortification of dry-packed cereals.

TABLE 2. *Iron absorption from infant foods*

Food	Forti- fication iron	Number of infants	Iron (mg) in test meal	[58]Fe incorporation (% of dose)	
				Geometric mean	±1 SD range
Rice cereal with apples and bananas	$FeSO_4$	12	2.8	5.4	2.9–10.0
Rice cereal with formula	$FeSO_4$	9	1.1	4.4	1.6–11.9
Vegetables and beef	$FeSO_4$	10	3.2	2.5	1.2– 5.3
Grape juice	$FeSO_4$	10	2.8	4.8	2.1–11.1
Rice cereal with formula	Fe fumarate	9	4.6	4.0	2.5–6.5

From ref. 5.

CONCLUSION

The use of stable isotopes now offers an approach to the assessment of iron bioavailability in normal infants and young children, the group at greatest risk of iron deficiency. Results in these initial studies generally agree with results from studies with radioisotopes. In the only previous study on iron absorption from infant foods, Rios et al. (6), using whole body counting after administration of radioiron (^{59}Fe), found that the geometric mean absorption of ferrous sulfate fed with mixed grain infant cereal was 2.7%. Thus, stable isotope studies can now be used to obtain information on the bioavailability of iron from infant foods.

REFERENCES

1. Bothwell, T. H., Charlton, R. W., Cook, J. D., and Finch, C. A. (1979): *Iron Metabolism in Man.* Blackwell Scientific Publications, Oxford.
2. Janghorbani, M., Ting, B. T. G., and Fomon, S. J. (1986): Erythrocyte incorporation of ingested stable isotope of iron (^{58}Fe). *Am. J. Hematol.*, 21:277.
3. Fomon, S. J., Janghorbani, M., Ting, B. T. G., et al. (1988): Erythrocyte incorporation of ingested 58-iron by infants. *Pediatr. Res.*, 24:20.
4. Heinrich, H. C. (1970): Intestinal iron absorption in man—methods of measurement, dose relationship, diagnostic and therapeutic applications. In: *Iron Deficiency*, edited by L. Hallberg, H.-G. Harworth and A. Vannotti. Academic Press, London, New York, pp. 213-294.
5. Fomon, S. J., Ziegler, E. E., Rogers, R. R., et al. (1989): Iron absorption from infant foods. *Pediatr. Res.* (in press).
6. Rios, E., Hunter, R. E., Cook, J. D., Smith, N. J., and Finch, C. A. (1975): The absorption of iron as supplements in infant cereal and infant formulas. *Pediatrics,* 55:686.

Dietary Iron: Birth to Two Years,
edited by L. J. Filer, Jr.
Raven Press, Ltd., New York © 1989.

Discussion

Dr. Filer: How was the iron dose administered?

Dr. Ziegler: It was given through a nipple. The nipple was placed in the infant's mouth and 5 ml of solution was given slowly through the nipple and then flushed. We were very careful to administer the dose quantitatively.

Dr. Filer: How did you decide to use 80 mg of ascorbic acid?

Dr. Ziegler: We used enough ascorbic acid to get a high molar ratio of ascorbic acid to iron of about 14. This is not unlike what is done in studies using radioisotopes. It does not make any difference exactly how much ascorbic acid is given as long as it is the same every time.

Dr. Oski: In your stable isotope studies comparing the different foods, did all of the subjects receive the same foods?

Dr. Ziegler: No, they were all different subjects. There were between 9 and 12 subjects per group.

Dr. Filer: Did you analyze the grape juice for its vitamin C content?

Dr. Ziegler: No, but the label stated its content as 31 mg/dl.

Dr. Filer: That means that it probably had double that amount.

Dr. Dallman: What was the cost of the isotope preparation per milligram?

Dr. Ziegler: A stable isotope-enriched preparation costs about $100.00 per milligram.

Dr. Oski: Were these children fasting before the test dose was administered?

Dr. Ziegler: No. They were brought from home to the metabolic unit. Approximately 2 hr after their morning formula feeding, they received the test dose and then nothing for 2 hr.

Dr. Dallman: The variability in your study is actually not more than what is observed in radioisotope studies.

Dr. Ziegler: That is right. However, in radioisotope studies the variability can be reduced by giving a reference isotope.

Dr. Filer: Apparently, between 140 and 168 days of age there is not a very large change in the circulating ^{58}Fe: ^{57}Fe ratio. Have you considered giving another dose of ^{58}Fe enriched food to that same infant using ^{58}Fe as a reference standard and just enriching it?

Dr. Ziegler: You could do that, but the second dose would need to be administered at least 2 weeks later, and during that time the physiological state of the infant could change. Technically, it could be done. I do not know whether that would solve the problem. We have not tried it.

Dietary Iron: Birth to Two Years,
edited by L. J. Filer, Jr.
Raven Press, Ltd., New York © 1989.

Nutritional Sources of Iron in Infants and Toddlers

Philip A. Walravens

Department of Pediatrics, University of Colorado Health Sciences Center, Denver, Colorado 80262

In this review, dietary sources of iron during infancy will be discussed briefly, and emphasis will be placed on sources of dietary iron for toddlers. In a recent study in Denver (unpublished), we found an unexpected incidence of iron depletion and deficiency in 18- to 24-month-old toddlers from low-income families. Nutrient analysis revealed that dietary iron intake was limited in these children. A subsample of these children was given a low-dose iron supplement, and a repeat assessment of iron nutriture was performed 6 months later. In this review, the nutritional and laboratory data collected in Denver will be compared with that collected in Scandinavian and North and Central American countries.

DIETARY IRON IN INFANCY: BIRTH THROUGH 12 MONTHS

For breast-fed infants, the elegant studies of Siimes et al. (1) showed that 33 solely breast-fed infants could maintain an adequate iron nutritional status until 6 months of age. The maintenance of an adequate iron status during this period of rapid growth demonstrates the excellent bioavailability·of iron from human milk. However, if human milk continues to be the major source of nutrients for longer than 6 months, an iron supplement must be provided.

DIETARY SOURCES OF IRON SUPPLEMENTS

Among formula-fed infants, the majority will receive cow's milk–based products, which are generally supplemented with 12 mg of iron/liter. Providing such products over the first 12 months of life insures both adequate iron nutrition and the establishment of reserves. Since iron deficiency in infancy may be related to the early provision of cow's milk (2), it is of some concern that the American Academy of Pediatrics in 1983 sanctioned the introduction of whole cow's milk at 6 months of age for infants who were receiving at least 30% of their diets as mixed solids (3). This concern is supported by the observations of Tunnessen and Oski (4), who showed that infants fed cow's milk at 6 months had, by 12 months of age, diminished reserves and a higher incidence of iron deficiency and lower hemoglobin values than formula-fed controls. The deficiencies occurred even though iron-fortified cereals were provided to many children receiving whole cow's milk. The study on intestinal blood loss by Ziegler in this volume provides additional support for continued feeding of iron-fortified formula in the latter half of the first year of life.

Another often-encountered practice consists of giving formulas low in iron because of concerns over gastrointestinal upsets associated with iron-fortified cow's milk products. The problems are generally described as a combination of frequent spitting up, cramping, and hard stools.

In a controlled study by Nelson and colleagues (5), the only demonstrable difference between infants fed the iron-fortified or low-iron cow's milk formula was the color of stools, which were more often dark brown, green, or black in the iron-supplemented group. Since pediatricians at times are obliged to give into parental wishes, a reasonable approach would be to permit a low-iron formula during the first 2 to 3 months of life when neonatal iron reserves are being mobilized. Later, iron-supplemented formula should be strongly recommended.

The study from Chile by Hertrampf and colleagues is reassuring to physicians who have prescribed soy-based formula products for those infants who cannot tolerate cow's milk (6). Good levels of hemoglobin and other indicators of iron status were present at 9 months of age in 47 infants who received soy formula for a period of 6 to 7 months. A 27% incidence of anemia was found, however, in a breast-fed group that served as the control. Although soy formula has long been considered to inhibit iron absorption, increased ascorbic acid concentration in the formula may compensate for the less favorable properties of a soy protein isolate.

EFFECT OF IRON-FORTIFIED CEREALS ON IRON NUTRITURE

There is some evidence that solid foods or infant cereals fortified with iron do little to improve iron status. Anemia was a frequent finding in the Chilean breast-fed infants, although solid foods were introduced at 3 to 4 months of age (6). Similarly, in the Syracuse study (4), 91% of infants fed whole cow's milk were eating fortified cereal at 8 months of age. By 12 months, 62% of the infants were still taking iron-supplemented cereals, but this practice did little to improve their hematological status. Whether this results from mixing fortified cereal with cow's milk and formation of iron phosphate–insoluble complexes remains unknown.

IRON-FORTIFIED CEREALS AND IMPROVED
BIOAVAILABILITY

The fortification of cereals and infant foods was discussed by Rees et al. in 1985 (7). Compared to one decade earlier (Table 1), the use of iron compounds of low bioavailability had markedly decreased by 1982. Infant cereals may now be fortified to levels of 13.5 mg of iron/ounce. Ferric phosphate salts at the time were found only in regular, not infant, cereals.

The benefits of providing iron-supplemented formulas and cereals for low income groups have been described for recipients of the Special Supplemental Food Program for Women, Infants, and Children (WIC) (8,9). In a study in New Haven, Connecticut, the mean hemoglobin level of 324 children enrolled in the WIC program who were followed at an inner city health center was 0.7 g/dl higher in 1984 than in 1971 (8). Similarly, Miller and colleagues (9), in a retrospective analysis of 1977 data from Minneapolis, showed that participation in the WIC program caused significant improvement of iron reserves in infants and a lesser incidence of low hematocrit and iron depletion in toddlers.

The subjects of fortification and bioavailability have been reviewed by Dallman (10), whose suggestions to improve iron nutrition in weanlings include increased use of ascorbic acid-enriched foods or juices and mixing meats with other solid foods after 6 months of age. However, it may be more practical to consider iron supplements for term infants when particular feeding practices are encountered. During the first 3 months of life, mobilization of iron from neonatal reserves is sufficient to cover needs. Thereafter, depending on the type of formula or milk provided, supplementation at a dose of 10 to 15 mg of iron daily should be considered for the later quartiles of the first year (Table 2).

TABLE 1. *Bioavailability of forms of iron used in cereal fortification: changes between 1972 and 1982*

	Iron bioavailability (%)	
	High[a]	Low[b]
1972		
Infant cereals	50	50
Cereal-based infant foods	60	40
Cereals	65	35
1982		
Infant cereals	100	–
Cereal-based infant foods	100	–
Cereals	88	12

[a]High bioavailability: iron sulfate, small particle reduced iron, iron fumarate.
[b]Low bioavailability: large particle reduced iron, iron phosphate salts.
[c]Adapted from ref. 7 with permission, J.B. Lippincott Co., © 1985.

The iron needs of premature infants are quite different and vary with birth weight and the degree of prematurity. Generally, after the second month, supplementation at a dose of 2 to 4 mg/kg/day is recommended (11).

DIETARY IRON IN THE TODDLER YEARS: THE DENVER STUDY OF CHILDREN IN LOW-INCOME HOUSEHOLDS

This project was designed to determine the effect of a multivitamin supplement containing iron and zinc on hematological parameters, plasma zinc concentration, dietary intake, growth rate, and developmental performance. Infants enrolled in the study received their routine pediatric care at the Westside Health Center in Denver, a clinic that primarily serves low-income families.

Recruitment was aimed at toddlers who were 18 to 24 months of age at the start of the 6-month observation and follow-up period. A large poster with sign-up sheets was placed in the entry hall of the Clinic, where about 15,000 pediatric encounters occur annually. Recruitment was generally voluntary. As an additional incentive, a stipend of $45 was offered to those who completed all aspects of the study. Of the first 190 subjects who entered the study, 140 (74%) completed the project. The data discussed in this chapter concern this group only.

An additional 40 subjects participated in the program; however, they were recruited by telephoning those families with children whose immunization schedules were up to date. Compliance was markedly better in this group, as 35 (87.5%) of the children completed the project. Dietary data were not collected for these children because the emphasis was mainly on growth velocity; for 12 of the 40 children, finger sticks only were performed upon the first visit.

Subjects were randomly assigned to one of five groups: (a) a plain multivitamin tablet (MV), (b) the same multivitamin with 12 mg of iron (MV + iron), (c) a multivitamin with iron and 8 mg of zinc (MV + minerals), (d) a multivitamin with 8 mg of zinc (MV + zinc), or (e) a placebo. The sup-

TABLE 2. *Feeding practices and supplemental iron needs in term infants*

	0–3 months	4–6 months	7–9 months	10–12 months
Breast milk	–	–	+	+
Cow's milk formula				
(low iron)	–	+	+	+
Iron enriched	–	–	–	–
Soy formula	–	–	–	–
Cow milk	–	+	+	+

Plus sign indicates the need for supplemental iron.

plements were provided in two batches of 100 tablets each, and compliance was assessed by counting the remaining pills at the 3- and 6-month visits. Families were instructed to provide one tablet daily, and follow-up visits were scheduled 3 and 6 months after the start of the study.

At the first visit, after anthropometric measurements were obtained, the child was tested with the Bayley Scales of Infant Development, and the caregivers were instructed to keep diet records. A venipuncture was attempted, and if it was successful, the following assays were performed: plasma zinc, hematological panel with indices (CBC), zinc protoporphyrin (ZPP), and serum ferritin. With small volumes, only ZPP, CBC, and plasma zinc levels were measured. If venipuncture failed, or if the parents objected, a capillary finger stick was used to obtain a hematological panel.

At the 3- and 6-month visits, anthropometric tests, developmental tests, and diet record collection were repeated. Venipuncture was repeated at the end of the 6-month study.

With regard to the laboratory assays, normal values included a hemoglobin concentration greater than 11.2 g/dl, zinc protoporphyrin levels less than 40 µg/dl, serum ferritin greater than 20 ng/ml, and mean corpuscular volume greater than 70 fl. Iron depletion was considered if serum ferritin levels alone were decreased. Iron deficiency can manifest itself by biochemical changes including microcytosis before anemia appears. In iron deficiency with anemia, hemoglobin levels are decreased, zinc protoporphyrin concentrations are elevated, and serum ferritin levels are low.

Seventy-two-hour diet record collection was also part of this study, and at the initial interview, the caregivers were instructed on proper methods of keeping diet records. The records were examined for completeness and accuracy first by a child health associate and later by a nutritionist. The actual analysis was performed by graduate students in nutrition from Cornell University under the supervision of Dr. Diva Sanjur. Complete food records were provided by 78 subjects, while an additional 12 provided at least one record from each study period. A total of 793 records from 90 subjects were the basis for the final analysis, for 72% of the total 1,104 diet records obtained during the investigation.

DEMOGRAPHIC AND SOCIOECONOMIC CHARACTERISTICS OF THE DENVER TODDLERS

Of 90 children, 67% were Hispanic, 31% were white, and 2% were black. Although yearly income ranged from $3,264 to $35,000, 34% of the participant families had incomes of less than $5,000 a year (Table 3), and 73% of the families fell below poverty limits. Educational levels of the mothers are summarized in Table 3. Regarding maternal occupations, 66 mothers were homemakers (72%), 20 were clerical, sales, manual, or skilled workers, and 4 were students. The mean family size was three members; only 10 families had more than five, and 30 had fewer than three members. Male heads of household were excluded from the computation of family size.

Of the first 190 subjects, hemoglobin levels were obtained on 179 children, and 12 had concentrations below 11.2 g/dl. Zinc protoporphyrin levels in excess of 40 µg/dl were present in 44 of 153 subjects, and serum ferritin levels were low in 39 of 140 samples. Because of problems with blood collection, sample size, and clotting, some assays were not done on all subjects.

Further analysis of these biochemical criteria provided a better definition of the iron nutritional status of the population upon entry to the study. Twenty-eight subjects had iron depletion alone with low serum ferritin levels, 42 had biochemical evidence of iron deficiency manifested by increases in zinc protoporphyrin concentration, and two subjects had iron deficiency with anemia. Ten subjects had infection-induced anemia, in which zinc protoporphyrin and serum ferritin levels were normal and the situation corrected spontaneously. There was no evidence of lead toxicity in the subjects with zinc protoporphyrin levels greater than 50 µg/dl. Hence, laboratory evidence of inadequate iron status was present in 72 of 190 (38%) of the participants at the beginning of the study.

Mean values for serum ferritin, before and after supplementation, are shown in Fig. 1. These results are grouped according to the supplement received. In the MV + iron group, mean serum ferritin levels appear to be increased after 6 months of supplementation; however, because of the variability in results, these differences were not significant. Since this was a longitudinal study, it provided the opportunity to compare differences in serum ferritin levels before and after 6 months of supplementation. In Fig. 2, these paired differences are summarized according to the various supple-

TABLE 3. *Annual household income and years of education of mothers of 90 children from low-income Denver families*

	Number (N = 90)	Percent of sample
Annual household income ($)		
< 5,000	31	34
5,000–11,000	35	39
11,001–15,000	12	19
15,001–20,000	7	8
> 20,000	5	6
Education of mothers (years)		
College graduate (16)	4	5
Junior college		
(partial: 14)	15	17
High school graduate (12)	40	44
Some high school (10)	31	34

mentation groups. Positive mean differences in serum ferritin levels (ferritin at 6 months – ferritin at onset) were found only in the subjects receiving some form of iron supplement. Negative mean differences in serum ferritin occurred in the other three groups. There were significant differences in the paired mean changes in ferritin between the MV + iron group and three other groups (plain MV, MV + zinc, and placebo). There also was a trend toward significance between the MV + minerals and the plain MV, the MV + zinc, and placebo groups. No differences were evident between the MV + iron and the MV + minerals groups.

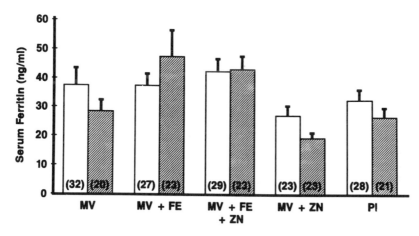

FIG. 1. Mean (SEM) serum ferritin concentrations before (open boxes) and after (hatched boxes) 6 months of supplementation with multivitamins or placebo. Sample size is indicated by numbers in parentheses within each bar.

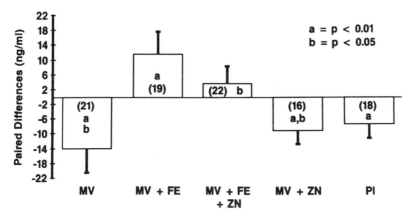

FIG. 2. Mean (SEM) paired differences in serum ferritin concentrations after 6 months of multivitamin or placebo supplementation. Number of subjects for whom paired samples were obtained is indicated in parentheses within each bar.

NUTRIENT AND ENERGY INTAKES OF CHILDREN IN THE DENVER STUDY

In general, nutrient and energy intakes were adequate (Table 4), and intakes of vitamin A, thiamine, riboflavin, and niacin (not included in Table 4) were all at or above the Recommended Dietary Allowances (12). Because of its potentiating effect on iron absorption, the daily intake of ascorbic acid was particularly critical. With regard to distribution of energy, protein intake averaged 15.3%, fat 34.3%, and carbohydrate 50.4% of total caloric intake. Iron was the most limiting nutrient, with a mean daily intake of 7.6 mg, which is 51% of the recommendation for this age group. The dietary intakes of magnesium (59% of RDA) and calcium (85% of RDA) were also inadequate. Of concern also were excessive intakes of potassium and sodium.

Analysis of iron intake by food group is show in Fig. 3. The cereal group was the largest contributor (40.4%), presumably because of fortification of breakfast cereals; the meat group (20.6%) and fruits (12.0%) also provided fair amounts of iron. According to the formulation of Monsen and colleagues (13), an easily absorbable iron level is 0.5 mg daily. Whenever cereals and dairy products contribute 50% or more of total energy intake, they become potential inhibitors of iron absorption. Thus, it is not surprising that iron depletion is a frequent finding in infancy.

OTHER STUDIES OF IRON NUTRITURE IN CHILDREN 18 TO 36 MONTHS OF AGE

A number of reports on iron nutriture among children 18 to 36 months of age have been carried out in the last 15 years (Table 5). Brault-Dubuc and colleagues in 1983 (14) presented an extensive report on iron intake in

TABLE 4. *Dietary intakes of 90 children from low-income Denver families (mean: ± SD)*

Nutrient	Intake	Range	% RDA
Energy (kcal)	1142 ± 327	483–2239	95
Protein (g)	45 ± 14	16–91	193
Fat (g)	45 ± 15	12–87	—
Carbohydrate (g)	146 ± 50	42–323	—
Iron (mg)	7.6 ± 2.6	3–16	51
Vitamin C (mg)	52 ± 42	2–136	117
Calcium (mg)	680 ± 379	145–2137	85
Magnesium (mg)	89 ± 42	7–206	59
Phosphorus (mg)	822 ± 420	261–2126	103
Sodium (mg)	1344 ± 507	523–2681	207
Potassium (mg)	1583 ± 542	427–3064	288

RDA, Recommended Dietary Allowance.

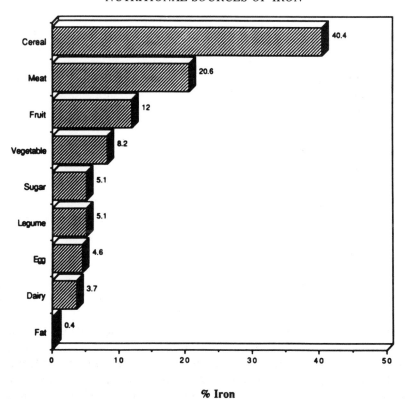

% Iron

FIG. 3. Mean contribution of various food groups to the daily dietary iron intake of 90 toddlers from low-income Denver families.

TABLE 5. *Dietary iron intake of children 18–36 months of age in seven worldwide studies*

City/country (ref.)	Mean intake (mg)			Income/area	Age (months)	Year of study
	All	Boys	Girls			
Denver (U.S.)[a]	7.6			Low/urban	18–24	Ongoing
Solis (Mex) (16)	11.2			Low/rural	18–30	Ongoing
Great Britain (19)		7.0	6.5	Mixed/mixed	24	1980
Manitoba (15)	7.9			Low/rural	35	1981
Montreal (14)		7.9	7.5	Medium/urban	24	1983
Finland (17)		10.0	9.0	Medium/mixed	36	1985
Sweden (18)		11.2	10.9	Medium/mixed	24	1986

[a]Present report.

Montreal infants from 3 to 36 months of age. In this longitudinal follow-up study of French Canadian middle-income families, the data collected between 1975 and 1979 included dietary intakes and laboratory assays of iron nutriture at quarterly intervals for children up to 24 months and again at 36 months of age. At 24 months, the median iron intake of the boys was 7.7 mg, ranging from 5.2 to 12.5 mg, or the 10th and 90th percentiles, respectively. Iron intakes of the female toddlers were slightly lower. Serum ferritin concentrations below 10 ng/ml, indicative of very poor reserves, were found in 7.8%, and low ferritin levels (10–20 ng/ml) occurred in 51.2% of the 166 2-year-old infants. At 24 months, the total incidence of hypoferritinemia was 59%, which decreased to 28.1% by 3 years of age.

In another Canadian study, toddlers from two isolated Indian villages in Manitoba were surveyed during the Winter, Spring, and Fall of 1974 (15). At a mean age of 35 months, more than one-half of the children were consuming less than the 7 to 9 mg of iron recommended by the Canadian Dietary Standards (15). Mean intakes in Winter and Spring approximated 8 mg/day and were lower than the mean intake in the fall, which reached 11 mg. In these villages, 33% to 42% of the ingested iron came from meat and alternative products, including fish, eggs, and legumes.

In a recent project, Allen and colleagues (L. H. Allen, personal communication) studied iron intake in toddlers (18–36 months) in the town of Solis, Mexico. The mean iron intake averaged 12.2 mg/day with a range from 6.7 to 20 mg, although only 0.2 mg was from animal sources. Heme iron ranged from 0.02 to 1.08 mg, compared to a mean intake of 1.85 of heme iron in NHANES II. Allen's observations are based on measurements performed 2 days/month over a 12-month period. Blood samples were collected in 39 children, and iron deficiency was present in one-third (16).

Two large nutritional surveys have recently been published from Scandinavia, where dietary records were generally collected between 1980 and 1981. Rasanen and colleagues (17) reported the results of the Finnish surveys compiled in 5 university cities and 12 surrounding rural communities. The mean iron intake for a group of 281 3-year-old children was 10 mg for the boys and 9 mg for the girls (SD of 4 mg). The relative contributions of meat products and cereals to the daily iron intake were 22% and 53%, respectively.

From Sweden, Hagman and colleagues (18) published the results of their childhood nutrient survey. Data were collected in Uppsala and Umea, two university and administrative centers and two rural areas. The mean intake of 2-year-old toddlers was 11.2 mg, with a range of 7.0 to 18 mg. Twenty-two percent of the Swedish toddlers were receiving less than 60% of the RDA. The contributions of meat products and cereals to the iron intake of the Swedish infants were 29% and 30%, respectively.

As Table 5 shows, the Denver toddlers were in the low ranges for dietary iron. The levels were similar to those documented in Great Britain, where mean iron intakes of 6.5–7 mg were found in a survey of 2-year-olds during the previous decade (19). Erhardt, however, recently documented iron deficiency anemia in 7% of white children and 21% of Asian children in Bradford (20); he suggested the need for a community-based preventive program. The Montreal study found a progressive increase in serum ferritin levels between 24 and 36 months in middle-class children. No such trend was present in the Denver study, since at completion of the 6-month observation period, 30% of the children still had ferritin levels less than 20 ng/ml.

Furthermore, in 56 subjects who received a multivitamin product containing iron and for whom we have initial and final hemoglobin levels, 10 increased their hemoglobin concentrations by more than 1 g/dl. Whether this relates to the supplemental iron, to lessened infection, or both remains to be determined, but it does appear that iron nutriture remains less than satisfactory in this low-income group.

In high-risk populations, a second screening of iron status should be performed in the toddler years, with the inclusion of zinc protoporphyrin levels to detect early iron deficiency. Another alternative would be to offer a 6-month period of low-dose iron supplementation if this can be done safely. The formulation used in the Denver study contained 1,200 mg of iron/bottle, which could be a dangerous dose if all of the tablets were consumed at once. Lesser risk would incur if chewable products containing iron supplements for children were provided in bottles holding only 30 or 50 tablets. In toddlers from disadvantaged families, improvements of iron nutriture should remain an objective of the medical and nutritional communities.

ACKNOWLEDGMENTS

This project was generously supported by a grant from the Mead Johnson Nutritionals. The encouragement and support of Dr. Angel Cordano and Dr. Duvi Carrera were much appreciated. The dietary data were analyzed by Ruth Aguilar, Alicia Garcia, and Molly Mort, nutrition students from Cornell University under the supervision of Dr. Diva Sanjur. Finally, this project could not have been completed without the help of the clerical, nursing, and clinical staff of the pediatric section at the Westside Health Center in Denver.

REFERENCES

1. Siimes, M. A., Salmenpera, L., and Perheentupa, J. (1984): Exclusive breast-feeding for nine months: risk of iron deficiency. *J. Pediatr.*, 104:196–199.
2. Sadowitz, P. D., and Oski, F. A. (1983): Iron status and infant feeding practices in an urban ambulatory center. *Pediatrics*, 72:33–36.
3. American Academy of Pediatrics Committee on Nutrition (1983): The use of whole cow's milk in infancy. *Pediatrics*, 72:253–255.

4. Tunnessen, W. W., and Oski, F. A. (1987): Consequences of starting whole cow milk at six months of age. *J. Pediatr.,* 111:813–816.
5. Nelson, S. E., Ziegler, E. E., Copeland, A. M., Edwards, B. B., and Fomon, S. J. (1988): Lack of adverse reactions to iron-fortified formula. *Pediatrics,* 81:360–364.
6. Hertrampf, E., Cayazzo, M., Pizarro, F., and Steckel, A. (1986): Bioavailability of iron in soy-based formula and its effect on iron nutriture in infancy. *Pediatrics,* 78:640–645.
7. Rees, J. M., Monsen, E. R., and Merrill, J. E. (1985): Iron fortification of infant foods. A decade of change. *Clin. Pediatr.,* 24:707–710.
8. Vazquez-Seoane, P., Windom, R., and Pearson, H. A. (1985): Disappearance of iron-deficiency anemia in a high-risk infant population given supplemental iron. *N. Engl. J. Med.,* 213:1239–1240.
9. Miller, V., Swaney, S., and Deinard, A. (1985): Impact of the WIC program on the iron status of infants. *Pediatrics,* 75:100–105.
10. Dallman, P. R. (1986): Iron deficiency in the weanling: a nutritional problem on the way to resolution. *Acta Pediatr. Scand.,* 323 (suppl):50–67.
11. Dallman, P. R. (1988): Nutritional anemia of infancy: iron, folic acid, and vitamin B12. In: *Nutrition During Infancy,* edited by R. C. Tsang and B. F. Nichols. Hanley & Belfus, Philadelphia, p. 225.
12. Food and Nutrition Board, National Research Council (1980): *Recommended Dietary Allowances.* National Academy of Sciences, Washington, D.C.
13. Monsen, E. R., Hallberg, L., Layrisse, M., Hegsted, D. M., Cook, J. D., and Mertz, W. (1978): Estimation of available dietary iron. *Am. J. Clin. Nutr.,* 31:134–141.
14. Brault-Dubuc, M., Nadeau, M., and Dickie, J. (1983): Iron status of French–Canadian children: a three-year follow-up. *Hum. Nutr. Appl. Nutr.,* 37A:210–221.
15. Ellestad-Sayet, J. J., Haworth, J. C., Coodin, F. J., and Dilling, L. A. (1981): Growth and nutrition of preschool Indian children in Manitoba: II. Nutrient intakes. *Can. J. Publ. Health,* 72:127–133.
16. Black, A. K., Allen, L. H., Mata, M., and Pelto, G. H. (1988): Dietary correlates of hematological status in Mexican preschoolers. *FASEB J.* 2:A1204.
17. Rasanen, L., Ahola, M., Kara, R., and Uhari, M. (1985): Atherosclerosis precursors in Finnish children and adolescents. VIII. Food consumption and nutrient intakes. *Act Paediatr. Scand.,* 318(suppl):135–153.
18. Hagman, U., Bruce, A., Persson, L. A., Samuelson, G., and Sjolin, S. (1986): Food habits and nutrient intake in childhood in relation to health and socioeconomic conditions. A Swedish multicentre study 1980–81. *Acta Paediatr. Scand.,* 328(suppl):4–56.
19. Darke, S., Disselduff, M., and Try, G. (1980): Frequency distributions of mean daily intakes of food energy and selected nutrients obtained during nutrition surveys of different groups of people in Great Britain between 1968 and 1971. *Br. J. Nutr.,* 44:243–252.
20. Ehrhardt, P. (1986): Iron deficiency in young Bradford children from different ethnic groups. *Br. Med. J.,* 292:90–93.

Dietary Iron: Birth to Two Years,
edited by L. J. Filer, Jr.
Raven Press, Ltd., New York © 1989.

Iron Nutrition: Growth in Infancy

George M. Owen

Medical Director, Bristol-Myers International Group,
New York, New York 10154

In evaluating iron nutrition and growth in infancy and early childhood, many variables should be taken into account: iron endowment at birth, rate of weight gain, blood loss, the level and bioavailability of iron in diet, postnatal age, and possibly sex and race.

Because of rapid growth and low body content of iron, the preterm infant requires more iron than the full-term infant. Iron requirements are greatest and iron deficiency is most prevalent during periods of rapid growth. The importance of growth is apparent from the age distribution of iron deficiency anemia. The increase in blood volume and red blood cell mass correlates with weight gain during infancy and childhood (1) (Fig. 1). Hence, the curve depicting annual increments in red blood cell mass and the curve depicting the distribution of iron deficiency anemia are similar. By redistributing iron and by lowering hemoglobin concentration, the healthy term infant is able to double its birth weight without requiring an exogenous iron source. For full-term infants, this doubling of birth weight occurs at 4 to 5 months of age. Thereafter, iron must be absorbed from the diet if supply is to meet demand. Siimes (2) asked the logical question: Are fast-growing, full-term infants at higher risk of developing iron deficiency than those who grow slowly, or do those who grow more rapidly absorb more iron?

In all studies examining nutritional status, blacks tend to be smaller than whites at birth. By 2 years of age, black children are taller, heavier, and thinner than white children (3) (Table 1). Black infants, who probably have less total body iron at birth, grow more rapidly and accumulate relatively more lean tissue (bone and muscle) and less fat than do white infants, while consuming less protein, iron, and ascorbic acid.

Black children tend to grow faster, and they have lower levels of hemoglobin than do white children of the same age, socioeconomic status, and transferrin saturation (4) (Table 2). Oski and Pearson (5) noted that black children with hemoglobin concentrations in the 10.5 to 11.0 g/dl range were four times more likely to have low mean corpuscular volume or ferritin and high free erythrocyte protoporphyrin levels than black children with hemo-

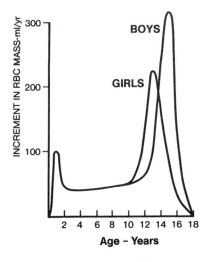

FIG. 1. Mean annual increment in red blood cell mass during childhood. Peaks in the curve correspond with peak periods in rate of growth and in the incidence of iron deficiency. (Reproduced from ref. 1 with permission from Harper and Row, © 1985.)

TABLE 1. *Anthropometric differences between black and white preschool boys of comparable socioeconomic status[a]*

Age interval (years)	Height (cm)	Weight (kg)	Skinfold (mm)
1.50–2.49	+ 1.29[b]	+ 0.37	− 0.09
2.50–3.49	+ 1.86[c]	+ 0.70[c]	− 0.29
3.50–4.49	+ 1.27	+ 0.48	− 0.37
4.50–5.49	+ 2.20[c]	+ 1.10[c]	− 0.45

[a]Adapted from ref. 3. (Reproduced with permission from the American Medical Association, © 1973.)
[b]Difference between black and white boys: black boys are 1.29 cm taller than white boys.
[c]Significant difference ($p < 0.05$).

TABLE 2. *Hemoglobin levels according to transferrin saturation, age, and race in preschool children of comparable socioeconomic status[a]*

| Age and race | Transferrin saturation | | |
	15–19%	20–24%	≥ 25%
24–47 months			
Black	118	121	129
White	126	125	128
48–71 months			
Black	118	125	123
White	128	130	130

Hemoglobin levels in g/liter.
[a]Adapted from ref. 4. (Reproduced with permission from the C. V. Mosby Co., © 1973.)

globin concentrations between 11.0 and 12.0 g/dl. They concluded that most children whose hemoglobin concentrations were between 10.5 and 11.0 g/dl had a nutritional basis for their mild anemia. Reeves et al. (6) also concluded that there was a nutritional basis for the difference in hemoglobin levels of black and white infants between 11 and 14 months of age. They found an equivalent response among both black and white infants following 3 months of treatment with iron (3 mg/kg/day), with 38% and 35%, respectively, manifesting an increase in hemoglobin concentrations of 1.0 g/dl or greater. It is of interest that in view of this similar response, these investigators concluded that black infants had a higher prevalence of iron deficiency.

Impaired growth has been attributed to anorexia, disturbances in nucleic acid synthesis, and altered small intestinal function associated with iron deficiency anemia. Naiman et al. (7) found decreased intestinal absorption of xylose and fat in infants with iron deficiency anemia. Iron deficiency that has progressed beyond depletion of iron stores (ferritin) will affect tissue iron compounds (heme iron compounds, and iron–sulfur and metallo-flavoproteins) and enzymes that do not contain iron but require it as a cofactor (8). Factors that play a role include the rate of tissue growth, turnover of individual iron compounds, and work load of individual tissues.

It is entirely possible that an infant's diet may be deficient in iron but otherwise nutritionally adequate, so that infants become sufficiently iron-deficient to impair growth. Yet, in reviewing the literature, it is difficult to determine at what point such an effect might be observed. It is clear that a number of factors contribute to the variability in observations regarding iron nutrition and growth, such as iron stores at birth, rate and possibly composition of growth, level and bioavailability of iron in diet, and losses of iron from body.

RETROSPECTIVE STUDIES

As iron deficiency develops, the rate of weight gain may decline; more severe iron deficiency and iron deficiency of longer duration may cause failure to thrive (8). Morton et al. (9) found that full-term infants with iron deficiency at age 12 months had a greater weight gain from birth than did iron-sufficient infants. They speculated that infants with greater weight gain had become iron-deficient from excessive demands for dietary iron.

Grindulis et al. (10) examined 145 children between 21 and 23 months of age: 55 (31%) had hemoglobin concentrations of less than 11.0 g/dl, and 25 (19%) had hemoglobin concentrations of less than 10.0 g/dl. Fifty-seven percent had plasma ferritin values of less than 7.0 ng/ml and transferrin saturation values of less than 15%. These investigators found no association between hemoglobin concentrations at age 22 months and body weight at birth or at 22 months (Table 3). They reported only mean values and appar-

TABLE 3. *Nutritional characteristics of Asian children at 22 months[a]*

	Hemoglobin (g/dl)		
	≥ 11.0	< 11.0	< 10.0
Body weight			
Birth (kg)	3.07	3.15	3.14
22 months (SDS[b])	+ 0.1	+ 0.3	+ 0.1

[a]Adapted from ref. 10. (Reproduced with permission from the *British Medical Journal,* © 1986.)
[b]Standard deviation scores.

ently did not evaluate separately children comprising the lower quartile with respect to hemoglobin concentration and weight gain from birth.

Owen et al. (11) found that preschool children whose heights for age were below the 25th percentile tended to have lower levels of hemoglobin and transferrin saturation than children whose heights were above the 25th percentile (Fig. 2). This was particularly true for children between 1 and 3 years of age.

Judisch et al. (12) reviewed medical records of 156 children (Fig. 3) less than 3 years of age who were diagnosed as having moderately severe iron deficiency anemia (hemoglobin < 9.0 g/dl, microcytosis and hypochromia, and low transferrin saturation). All infants were between 12 and 17 months of age when diagnosed, and one-third had a birth weight below 2,500 g. The majority (86%) were black. In 88 of 156 children, sufficient follow-up information was available to examine pre- and posttreatment body weights (6 mg of elemental iron/kg/day for 2 months). The frequency distribution of weights is shown in Fig. 4. It is evident that treatment with iron was associated with an improvement in weight.

A study of 10-month-old infants in two health districts in Paris (13) showed that plasma ferritin was low in 21%, and 12% of infants were anemic (hemoglobin < 11.0 g/dl). Apparent weight gain was inversely correlated with ferritin, suggesting a major effect of growth on iron metabolism (Table 4).

PROSPECTIVE STUDIES

Burman (14), in a study in Bristol (England), noted that birth weight was significantly related to hemoglobin concentration at age 3 months in boys only and at no other age. Among infants who did not receive supplementary iron, there was a slight sex difference in mean hemoglobin concentration; girls had a 0.4 g/dl greater concentration than boys at ages 15 and 18 months. The sex-related difference in hemoglobin concentration at these

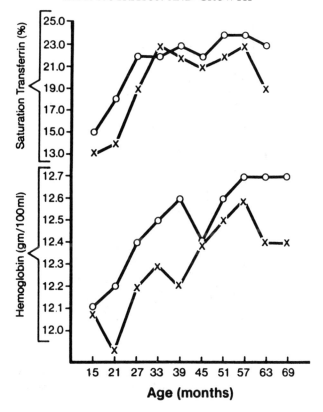

FIG. 2. Hemoglobin and transferrin saturation values in relation to age and stature. x = average hematological values of children whose heights were below the 25th percentile. ○ = values of children whose heights were equal to or above the 25th percentile. (Reproduced from ref. 11 with permission from the C. V. Mosby Co., © 1971.)

TABLE 4. *Ferritin concentration in relation to weight gain from birth to 10 months*[a]

	Weight gain (g)		
	< 5,000	5,000–6,500	>6,500
No. of infants	30	111	38
Birth weight (g)	3,360	3,220	3,140
Preterm (%)	7	8	21
Ferritin (μg/L)	26.9	21.7	17.3

[a]Adapted from ref. 13. (Reproduced with permission from the *Archives of French Pediatrics,* © 1984.)

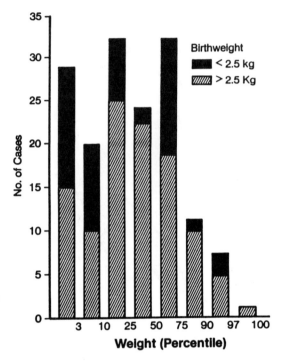

FIG. 3. Frequency distribution of weights at time of diagnosis of the entire group of 156 iron-deficient children. (Reproduced from ref. 12 with permission from *Pediatrics,* © 1966.)

ages may reflect the more rapid weight gain of boys during the first year of life.

Burman (15) randomly selected a cohort of infants at age 3 months to receive supplementary iron (10 mg daily), while the other infants received a placebo. In the placebo group, weight gain was significantly greater in boys than in girls at 3, 6, and 9 months. In the treatment group, weight gain was significantly greater in boys than in girls at 3, 6, 9, 12, 21, and 24 months. Weight gain was significantly greater in iron-supplemented than in non-iron-supplemented boys at ages 21 and 24 months. Iron supplementation had no significant effect on weight gain in girls at any age.

Among 470 children between 17 and 19 months of age in four health clinics in central Birmingham (England), 25% were found to have hemoglobin concentrations between 8.0 and 11.0 g/dl (16). Fifty-four children were treated with iron (24 mg) and vitamin C (10 mg) daily for 2 months, and 56 children received vitamin C only (10 mg daily) for the same period. Levels of hemoglobin and related hematological indices (mean corpuscular volume and mean corpuscular hemoglobin) as well as biochemical measures of iron nutriture (serum iron, transferrin saturation, and ferritin) all improved in the infants treated with iron but not in those treated with vitamin C alone. The

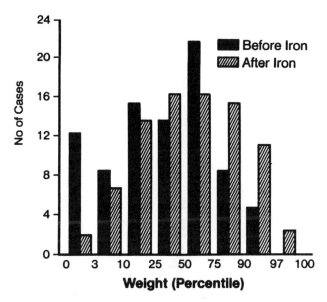

FIG. 4. Frequency distribution of weights of 88 iron-deficient children in whom follow-up data permitted comparison before and after iron therapy. (Reproduced from ref. 12 with permission from *Pediatrics,* © 1966.)

rate of weight gain in the children who received iron and vitamin C was 10 g/day, significantly greater than in those who received vitamin C only (7 g/day) (Fig. 5).

Chwang et al. (17) demonstrated improved growth in anemic (< 11.0 g/dl) and iron-deficient (transferrin saturation < 15%) school children who were treated with iron (2 mg/kg/day) for 12 weeks. Treatment effects were demonstrable for weight, height, and arm circumference in the anemic group but not in the nonanemic control group. Within the control group, no significant differences were seen between those who were treated with iron and those who received placebo.

In a longitudinal study of 276 full-term infants, all of whom stopped breast feeding by age 3 months, one-half received milk fortified with 3 mg of iron and 20 mg of ascorbic acid/100 kcal, and one-half received unfortified milk (18). Hematological data were comparable in the two groups at age 3 months. By age 9 months, the control group had significantly lower mean hemoglobin, transferrin saturation, serum ferritin, and elevated erythrocyte protoporphyrin (Fig. 6). Differences also existed at age 15 months (Fig. 7), although there were no differences in growth.

In a study of breast-fed and formula-fed infants, we examined iron nutriture and growth (19,20). Nearly equal numbers of male and female infants were present in each of four feeding groups: breast ($N = 26$), breast plus 10 mg/day of supplementary iron ($N = 27$), formula ($N = 41$), and iron-

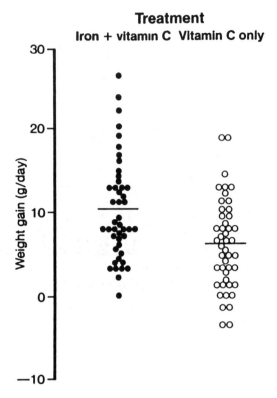

FIG. 5. Weight gain according to treatment group (*p* = 0.001). (Reproduced from ref. 16 with permission from the *British Medical Journal,* © 1986.)

fortified formula (*N* = 45) estimated to provide an intake of 10 mg of iron/day. Use of iron supplement or iron-fortified formula began when infants were 1 month of age. Formula-fed infants gained an average of 23.5 g/day, and breast-fed infants gained 19.3 g/day between 1 and 178 days of age. Within the breast-fed and formula-fed groups, there were no apparent differences in weight gain during the first 6 months to reflect iron supplementation (Table 5). The decrease in body storage iron (BSI) was greatest in the infants receiving formula and lowest in the infants in the breast plus supplementary iron group. The decrease in BSI was comparable in the other two groups, although infants in the group receiving iron-fortified formula gained weight at a significantly greater rate.

COMMENT

The Committee on Nutrition of the American Academy of Pediatrics suggests that determination of weight gain is the single most valuable component of the clinical evaluation of nutritional adequacy of the infant diet. A feeding-

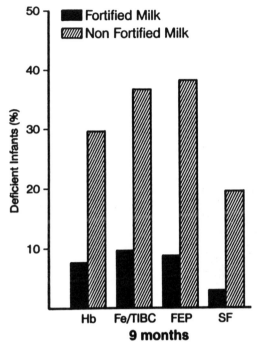

FIG. 6. Percentage of infants at 9 months of age with Hb < 110 g/liter, Fe/TIBC < 9%, FEP > 120 μg/dl (2.12 μmol/liter) of red blood cells, and SF < 10 μg/liter. (Reproduced from ref. 18 with permission from the *American Journal of Clinical Nutrition,* © 1988.)

related difference in weight gain of more than 3 g/day over a 3-month period during early infancy should be considered of nutritional significance.

If a sufficiently large group of infants were followed between 6 and 18 months of age, it is likely that slight changes in weight gain would be detected if biochemical changes indicative of iron depletion were found. It is reasonably certain that the rate of gain will decrease when the iron deficiency becomes severe and anemia is latent or actually developing. It is not possible to conclude whether the early phases of iron depletion are associated with an initial increase in rate of gain; this seems possible as the infant consumes more food than necessary, presumably in an effort to achieve an adequate iron intake.

TABLE 5. *Gain in body weight and decrease in body storage iron (BSI) from birth to 6 months in infants in four feeding groups*

Feeding group	Gain in weight (g/day)	Decrease in BSI (mg/kg)
Formula	+ 24.1	− 21.5
Iron-fortified formula	+ 23.0	− 18.9
Breast	+ 19.5	− 18.4
Breast + iron supplementation (10 mg/day)	+ 19.0	− 13.5

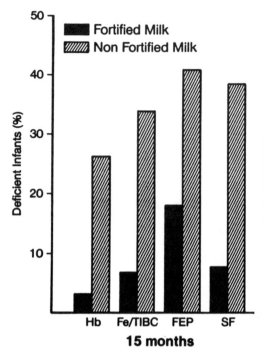

FIG. 7. Percentage of infants at 15 months of age with Hb < 110 g/liter, Fe/TIBC < 9%, FEP > 100 µg/dl (1.77 µmol/liter) of red blood cells, and SF < 10 µg/liter. (Reproduced from ref. 18 with permission from the *American Journal of Clinical Nutrition,* © 1988.)

REFERENCES

1. Lukens, J. N. (1985): Nutritional anemias in childhood. In: *Practice of Pediatrics,* revised ed., edited by V. C. Kelley. Harper and Row, Philadelphia.
2. Siimes, M. A. (1981): Pathogenesis of iron deficiency in infancy. In: *Iron Nutrition Revisited—Infancy, Childhood, Adolescence: Report of the 82nd Ross Conference on Pediatric Research,* edited by F. A. Oski and H. A. Pearson. Ross Laboratories, Columbus, pp. 96–108.
3. Owen, G. M., and Lubin, A. H. (1973): Anthropometric differences between black and white pre-school children. *Am. J. Dis. Child.,* 126:168–169.
4. Owen, G. M., Lubin, A. H., and Garry, P. J. (1973): Hemoglobin levels according to age, race and transferrin saturation in preschool children of comparable socioeconomic status. *J. Pediatr.,* 82:850–851.
5. Oski, F. A., and Pearson, H. A., eds. (1981): *Iron Nutrition Revisited—Infancy, Childhood, Adolescence: Report of the 82nd Ross Conference on Pediatric Research.* Ross Laboratories, Columbus, p. 42.
6. Reeves, J. D., Driggers, D. A., Lo, E. Y. T., and Dallman, P. R. (1981): Screening for anemia in infants: evidence in favor of using identical hemoglobin criteria for blacks and Caucasians. *Am. J. Clin. Nutr.,* 34:2154–2157.
7. Naiman, J. L., Oski, F. A., and Diamond, L. K. (1964): The gastrointestinal effects of iron defi-ciency anemia. *Pediatrics,* 33:83–99.
8. Oski, F. A. (1979): The non-hematologic manifestation of iron deficiency. *Am. J. Dis. Child.,* 133:315–322.
9. Morton, R. E., Nysenbaum, A., and Price, K. (1988): Iron status in the first year of life. *J. Pediatr. Gastroenterol. Nutr.,* 7:707–712.
10. Grindulis, H., Scott, P. H., Belton, N. R., and Wharton, B. A. (1986): Combined deficiency of iron and vitamin D in Asian toddlers. *Arch. Dis. Child.,* 61:843–848.
11. Owen, G. M., Lubin, A. H., and Garry, P. J. (1971): Preschool children in the United States: who has iron deficiency? *J. Pediatr.,* 79:563–568.

12. Judisch, J. M., Naiman, J. F., and Oski, F. A. (1966): The fallacy of the fat iron-deficient child. *Pediatrics,* 37:987–990.
13. Dommergues, J. P., Breton, M. P., Ducat, B., Yuart, J., Rossignol, C., and Tchernia, G. (1984): Carence en fer chez le nourrisson: étude des facteurs de risque. *Arch. Fr. Pediatr.,* 41:623–627.
14. Burman, D. (1972): Haemoglobin levels in normal infants aged 3–24 months, and the effect of iron. *Arch. Dis. Child.,* 47:261–271.
15. Burman, D. (1982): Iron deficiency in infancy and childhood. *Clin. Haematol.,* 11:339–351.
16. Aukett, M. A., Parks, Y. A., Scott, P. H., and Wharton, B. A. (1986): Treatment with iron increases weight gain and psychomotor development. *Arch. Dis. Child.,* 61:849–857.
17. Chwang, L., Soemantri, A. G., and Pollitt, E. (1988). Iron supplementation and physical growth of rural Indonesian children. *Am. J. Clin. Nutr.,* 47:496–501.
18. Stekel, A., Olivares, M., Cayazzo, M., Chadud, P., Llaguno, S., and Pizarro, F. (1988): Prevention of iron deficiency by milk fortification. II. A field trial with a full-fat acidified milk. *Am. J. Clin. Nutr.,* 47:265–269.
19. Garry, P. J., Owen, G. M., Hooper, E. M., and Gilbert, B. A. (1981): Iron absorption from human milk and formula with and without iron supplementation. *Pediatr. Res.,* 15:822–828.
20. Owen, G. M., Garry, P. J., and Hooper, E. M. (1984): Feeding and growth of infants. *Nutr. Res.,* 4:727–731.
21. Roche, A. F., and Himes, J. H. (1980): Incremental growth charts. *Am. J. Clin. Nutr.,* 33:2041–2052.

Dietary Iron: Birth to Two Years,
edited by L. J. Filer, Jr.
Raven Press, Ltd., New York © 1989.

Discussion

Dr. Filer: In the Albuquerque study, were there any differences in body length after 12 months?

Dr. Owen: I have only examined the weight data. There may be some subtle sex differences that affect nutritional needs for later growth. In the study by Walravens and Hambidge, there was a growth effect of zinc supplementation in male but not in female infants.

Dr. Filer: Do you have any information about the zinc status of these infants?

Dr. Owen: No.

Dr. Walravens: Individual variability makes it difficult to do studies of this type. Did you control for parental size? If you have many short parents, you will have many little children by age 9 to 12 months when the growth rate is slowing down due to influence on genetic growth potential.

Dr. Owen: The altitude in Albuquerque is about 5,500 ft (1,700 m) above sea level. Approximately 70% of the children were Hispanic. We do have height information for the mothers; however, I do not know if we have paternal heights. All infants were full-term and all were enrolled in the study prenatally. Parents were contacted sometime during the second or third trimester of pregnancy.

Dr. Oski: We have observed that as many children became iron-deficient, they begin to show a pattern of "failure to thrive."

Dr. Walravens: Are these children older?

Dr. Oski: Actually, their growth rate began to decrease at 6 or 7 months of age.

Dr. Walter: We have observed the same thing. However, we think that it is related to zinc status because it also happens in breast-fed infants. Ten years ago, we studied three groups of infants. One group was fed iron-fortified milk that had been acidified and one group was given nonfortified cow's milk. The third group was given 150 mg of iron dextran intramuscularly at birth. These three groups were followed to 3, 9, and 15 months of age. There were large differences in the ferritin levels between the groups. Infants given the iron-fortified milk were not anemic at 3 or 9 months of age, and very few had anemia at 15 months. A difference that we don't know how to interpret, however, is that the infants who were given iron dextran at birth had higher hemoglobin levels than those fed iron-fortified formula by 3 months of age. Very few of the infants in the iron dextran group had anemia at 9 months, and the incidence of anemia was comparable to that of infants fed the iron-fortified milk at 15 months. In the non-iron-fortified milk group, about 25% had anemia. The body weight of infants fed the non-iron-fortified milk was less than that of infants fed the iron-fortified formula. We believe that this difference has nothing to do with iron. At 3 months of age, all infants were well nourished according to their weight for age, but at 9 and 15 months, their mean growth curve fell off although they remained within the normal range. We believe that this difference in body weight occurred because infants in the iron-fortified formula group drank more milk and grew better. The fortified formula also had additional vitamins A and D that were not added to the nonfortified milk. There was no difference in mean body weight for age between the iron dextran and non-iron-fortified milk groups even though there was a large difference in iron status. These same relationships between groups were observed for length for age. The linear growth curves of the iron–dextran and non-iron-fortified milk groups were the same with linear growth of the iron-fortified milk group somewhat higher than the other two groups. The falloff in the linear growth curve was more marked than the falloff in body weight, which is why we believe it is a zinc-related phenomenon. Also, male infants were more affected than female infants.

Dr. Filer: Why do you say this is a zinc effect?

Dr. Walter: We have serum zinc data and 60% of the infants who were being breast-fed exclusively or were being fed cow's milk have levels lower than 60 µg/dl at 9 months of age. All samples were obtained in the fasting state before 10:00 A.M.

Dr. Filer: How can you conclude that it is zinc that is having an effect?

Dr. Walter: I am only suggesting that. Our current study will provide conclusions.

Dr. Dallman: I find it difficult to come to grips with the topic as a whole because it seems to me that it can be broken down into several issues. For example, we know that birth weight is a major factor and that low-birth-weight infants, with their low iron stores, get iron-deficient early.

Dr. Owen: Of course, and, at the same time, the low-birth-weight infant is growing rapidly.

Dr. Dallman: Exactly. So, growth rate and iron deficiency are going to be linked in that the fastest-growing infants are the ones with the lowest birth weight and are also the ones who will get iron-deficient.

Dr. Oski: No one has ever done a study of iron-deficient infants who remain untreated to see what the rate of growth is.

Dr. Dallman: I agree. If one cancels out the birth weight issue, there may be two different situations going on. What Marty Siimes tried to assess was whether infants who had average birth weights but were very big at 1 year of age would have higher iron requirements than infants who started out larger at birth but did not gain very much during the first year. I believe that he made some hypothetical calculations of the iron requirement during the first year of life for fast- and slow-growing infants. It makes sense to me that the fastest-growing infant who has a higher iron requirement would be more vulnerable for iron deficiency. The other situation—the one that Dr. Oski may have observed—is that those infants who became iron deficient in early life may have a growth deficit at about the same time.

Dr. Oski: Iron-deficient infants actually become anorectic.

Dr. Dallman: It is difficult to pull all of these factors together because there are at least three separate issues. One of them is related to birth weight and the rate of growth due to prematurity; the second issue is that rapid growth is a causative factor in iron deficiency, as observed in adolescents; and the third issue is that an established iron deficiency has an influence on growth. If we could separate these issues, we could probably learn more about the pathophysiology of iron deficiency.

Dr. Oski: One of the best situations to observe the effects of rapid growth is in exclusively breast-fed babies. Those infants who grow most rapidly on human milk are the ones who are most likely to become iron-deficient.

Dr. Walter: I disagree, based on my serum zinc data from breast-fed infants at 9 months of age.

Dr. Filer: Actually, this situation may apply to any mineral deficiency. The faster the infant grows, the more likely it is that the infant will develop a deficiency. For example, this effect has been observed in copper deficiency.

Dietary Iron: Birth to Two Years,
edited by L. J. Filer, Jr.
Raven Press, Ltd., New York © 1989.

Iron and Infection

Tomas Walter, Manuel Olivares, and Fernando Pizarro

*Institute of Nutrition and Food Technology, University of Chile,
15138 Santiago 11, Chile*

The interaction between host and infectious agent is a complex phenomenon, and no theory or experimental model has encompassed that complexity. The central focus of scientific inquiry should be to identify the basic processes and factors of both the human immune response and infectious agent virulence. When reviewing the literature on the relationship of iron deficiency to infection, one encounters conflicting data and divergent results. Some investigators favor the contention that mild iron deficiency is "good" for immunity, while others contend that any iron deficit is not good for immunity.

To examine this controversy, we will address (a) the relationship of iron to the immune response *in vitro;* (b) the evidence that administration of iron may promote infection; (c) evidence that iron may protect against infection; (d) the effect of parenteral iron therapy; and (e) the effect of iron-fortified foods on infection during infancy.

IMMUNE RESPONSE *IN VITRO*

Two immune system abnormalities associated with iron deficiency have been documented in humans: an impaired response of T-lymphocytes to mitogens and a decreased bactericidal activity of neutrophils. The DNA synthesis of T-lymphocytes in response to stimulants or mitogens results in "blastic transformation" and the production of lymphokines that are important for immune regulation. A continuous supply of iron is required for the activity of mammalian ribonucleotide reductase (1), an obligatory step in DNA synthesis (2).

Joynson et al. (3) described an impairment in lymphocyte transformation and production of migration inhibition factor after *Candida* and purified protein derivative (PPD) antigen stimulation in 12 subjects with iron deficiency anemia. Both the proportion and absolute number of T-lymphocytes were reduced in iron deficiency anemia. Lymphocyte proliferation and response to phytohemagglutinin (PHA) and Con A antigens were impaired in iron deficiency without anemia, and there was a significant correlation between the stimulation index and transferrin saturation (4–6). In a recent study of 10 iron-deficient children aged 12 to 30 months, the mean stimulation index for *Candida* antigen increased from 6.8% to 17.9%, and for tetanus antigen from 19.5% to 31.7%, following iron therapy (7).

A defect in neutrophil function in iron-deficient patients could also predispose them to bacterial infection. Although it is generally agreed that phagocytosis, or ingestion of bacteria, is normal in the presence of iron deficiency (8–10), the capacity for killing certain types of bacteria once they have been ingested is impaired (11–13). At least two or three iron-dependent steps are involved in intracellular bacterial killing. A sharp increase in oxygen consumption or the "respiratory burst" (14) results from the activation of NADPH oxidase (presumably an iron–sulfur enzyme), which produces O_2 and H_2O_2. The heme protein cytochrome b is also associated with the "respiratory burst" in a way yet to be clarified. H_2O_2 and O_2 are used to produce oxidized halogens and $OH-$ radicals, which are effective in bacterial killing. The heme-iron enzyme myeloperoxidase mediates the halogenation of bacterial protein using H_2O_2. The production of OH-radicals is catalyzed by the iron present in leukocyte lactoferrin by way of the Haber–Weiss reaction (15).

Neutrophil function defects have been demonstrated *in vitro* for humans by Chandra. Walter et al. (16) have studied neutrophil function in 10 iron-deficient but otherwise healthy infants 6 to 23 months of age. Neutrophil function and iron status were assessed at 0, 3 to 5, 15, 30, and 90 days after oral iron therapy had been initiated. Although phagocytosis was unaffected, bactericidal activity was profoundly impaired before therapy, improved partially at 3 to 5 days, and was completely corrected at 15 days. The timing of recovery suggested that iron had no effect upon circulating neutrophils but was required for neutrophil development in the bone marrow. This finding is in accordance with the rate of recovery of myeloperoxidase activity in iron-deficient rats. In these iron-deficient rats, however, the "oxidative burst" was maintained, allowing other bacterial killing mechanisms to continue (17). This finding in the animal model may explain why no overt clinical signs (respiratory, gastrointestinal, or cutaneous) could be identified in this group of children either before they were studied or during the subsequent 15 days of close clinical and laboratory follow-up, in spite of profound *in vitro* immune defects. The clinical significance of these laboratory findings of immune function defects in moderately to severely iron-deficient infants is questionable.

The preceding studies provide convincing evidence of an unfavorable effect of iron deficiency on human T-cell and phagocyte function *in vitro*. In addition, bacteria require iron for growth, and increased iron availability enhances bacterial virulence. In fact, iron is avidly bound by bacterial iron transport cofactors called siderophores. The iron-binding affinity of siderophores is comparable to that of transferrin. Several *in vitro* experiments have shown that the addition of unsaturated transferrin or iron chelators such as desferroxamine to culture media inhibits bacterial growth and bacteria resume growth with iron replacement (18).

Less iron is available to bacteria during an infectious process due to the "iron shift" that occurs as part of the acute-phase reaction. The iron shift involves a rapid decrease in serum iron concentration with a consequent fall in transferrin saturation (19). Unsaturated transferrin could compete for available iron sources and contribute to an inhibition of microbial growth and decrease in virulence.

EVIDENCE THAT IRON MAY PROMOTE INFECTION

Over 100 years ago, Trousseau (20) observed that iron supplementation of patients with quiescent tuberculosis often led to clinical recurrence. McFarlane et al. (21) suggested that the rapid deterioration and death of infants with kwashiorkor was related to refeeding, especially micronutrient supplements containing iron. A direct correlation between serum transferrin concentration and survival was observed in a group of 40 children treated with a high protein diet, antimalarial agents, vitamins, and iron. Overwhelming infection was the most frequent cause of death. After 2 weeks of treatment, the mean serum transferrin concentration of those who survived was 130 mg/dl versus 30 mg/dl in those who did not survive. Serum albumin concentrations were also lower in those who died. Serum from infants dying of infection supported growth of *Staphylococcus aureus,* whereas the addition of purified transferrin to the cultures inhibited bacterial growth (22). McFarlane and co-workers suggested that in patients with low serum transferrin concentrations, iron therapy resulted in a high percent transferrin saturation that promoted bacterial infection. However, another explanation for these findings is that those who died had more severe kwashiorkor, as indicated by low serum transferrin and albumin concentrations.

The studies by Murray et al. (23–25) are widely quoted as evidence for a protective effect of iron deficiency on infection. In a prospective randomized trial of 137 adult Somali nomads with iron deficiency anemia, only patients with an otherwise normal nutritional status were enrolled. These subjects were given 900 mg of oral ferrous sulfate or a placebo for 1 month. Iron treatment raised serum iron and hemoglobin concentrations. In the untreated group ($n = 71$), there were 3 episodes (7.6%) of infection, compared with 36 episodes in 27 subjects (38%) in the iron-supplemented group ($n = 66$). Differences in rates of infection were noted for malaria, brucellosis, and tuberculosis. Although this study has been criticized because the follow-up time was limited and the study was not double-blinded, it is the most convincing evidence that oral iron treatment may increase the incidence of certain infectious illnesses.

EVIDENCE THAT IRON MAY PROTECT AGAINST INFECTION

In 1928, Mackay reported the results of a survey of 541 nonhospitalized infants in London (26). She observed that anemia was common in breast-fed and cow's milk–fed infants. Oral iron supplementation not only raised hemoglobin, but allegedly reduced the incidence of respiratory and diarrheal disease by 50%, compared to untreated controls. Unfortunately, important intervening variables were not reported. Furthermore, the study compared successive years of treated and untreated populations, instead of concurrently treated and untreated groups. However, it is remarkable that Mackay recommended 60 years ago that formula-fed infants be given an iron supplement before 2 months of age and that many breast-fed infants also require iron treatment.

Twenty years ago, Andelman and Sered (27) described the effect of feeding an iron-fortified formula for 6 to 9 months to 603 infants of low socio-economic status in Chicago and compared the results to 445 control infants fed a non-iron-fortified evaporated milk formula. Although growth was similar in both groups, 9% of the iron-treated infants had anemia compared to 76% of the untreated infants. There was also a striking reduction in the incidence of respiratory infection in the group receiving iron-fortified formula. This study has been criticized for the loose criteria defining infection and for the dependence on parental recall of illness. The same criticisms apply to a study by Burman (28) in which infants 3 to 24 months of age were randomized to receive iron or no supplementation with no difference in infection found between groups. Lovric (29) found that anemic children had a significantly higher prevalence of gastroenteritis than nonanemic controls. However, it is unclear whether the gastroenteritis is the cause or consequence of the anemia. Another study of Maori infants showed that infants who received parenteral iron dextran in the neonatal period had lower hospital admission rates during the subsequent 2 years, principally for some respiratory and gastrointestinal infections, than untreated controls (30). Randomization of infants as well as the selection of clinical end points were probably inadequate. Hospital admissions are not always based on standardized criteria, and these in turn may change over time.

Mucocutaneous candidiasis in pediatric and adult patients, associated with an iron deficit, improved when iron was administered (31,32). However, other studies have failed to show that iron status or treatment had a significant impact on either oral or genital candidiasis (33).

Oppenheimer et al. (34) showed in a retrospective study that meningitis and pneumonia were more common in the presence of iron deficiency in hospitalized infants in Papua New Guinea. However, the effect of infection on iron status measurements is now known to be a confounding factor when attempting to establish a relationship between iron status and infection after infection has occurred. The knowledge that alterations in iron status, which mimic iron deficiency anemia, may last several days or weeks after an acute infectious episode has subsided should give us a new perspective for evaluating past and future studies (19).

PARENTERAL IRON THERAPY

Barry and Reeve (32,35) have reported the results of giving a large number of Polynesian neonates prophylactic intramuscular iron dextran. During a 2-year period, the incidence of neonatal sepsis (usually due to *E. coli*) was 22 per 1,000 infants. After discontinuing the administration of iron dextran, the incidence of sepsis decreased to 1.8 per 1,000 infants. Most infections occurred 4 to 10 days after the injection without evidence of localized infection at the injection site. Several flaws in this study detract from the authors' conclusion that iron treatment was related to the increased incidence of death from sepsis. Rates of infection prior to the use of iron dextran were not provided, and since the entire population was treated, there were no simultaneous controls. Also, it is not clear whether the iron itself or the parenteral iron dextran was responsible for the effect. Unfortunately, once this paper was published, ethical issues precluded the study of the use of parenteral iron in neonates; thus, a well-planned study could not be carried out to clarify this issue.

In contrast to the study of Barry and Reeve, no increase in susceptibility to infection was seen in a study in the U.S. in which premature infants received prophylactic iron dextran (36). Also, a Finnish study of premature infants showed markedly lower infection rates during the first 6 months of life in neonates given prophylactic iron dextran than in untreated controls (37). Additionally, before Barry and Reeve's study was published, we gave 150 mg of iron dextran to 500 newborns in a maternity hospital in Santiago, and no cases of severe infection were detected during the first 4 days of life. Unfortunately, since 10 infants were lost to follow-up, the data on infection rates were not published (M. Olivares, personal communication).

Recently, a more extensive and carefully designed prospective, double-blind, longitudinal protocol has been carried out by Oppenheimer and co-workers in Madang, Papua New Guinea, where malaria is endemic (34,38). A total of 486 newborn infants were randomized to receive either 150 mg of elemental iron as intramuscular iron dextran or a placebo at 2 months of age. After 12 months of follow-up, death rates were similar in both groups, with the primary cause of death being lower respiratory infection related to measles or pertussis. However, in the iron-treated group, there was an increased incidence of otitis media, severe lower respiratory infections, malarial parasitemia, and splenomegaly rates. Hospital admissions associated with measles and malaria were also higher. After 6 months, 18.5% of the iron-treated group and 11.3% of controls were positive for malaria; and after 12 months, the percent positive were 33% and 20%, respectively. Nevertheless, no significant difference was found in the degree of parasitemia in the positive subjects. These carefully designed studies show that the difference in infection rates between iron-treated and non-iron-treated infants is at best marginal, except perhaps for malaria, a chronic disease for which infection rate and disease detectability are not synonymous. In the pathogenesis of malaria, a parasite that infects the red blood cell, newer erythrocytes are more susceptible to infection. Thus, it is conceivable that iron-deficient infants do not have as heavy parasitemia as the iron-replete infants and that actual infection rates are similar.

The contradictory findings reported in the literature on the interaction of iron and infection may be due to differences in the degree of exposure to infection. Most reports that support the concept of an increased risk of infection after iron treatment are based on studies of disadvantaged populations in developing tropical countries. In these populations, it is valid to assume that other nutritional deficits in addition to iron deficiency may be a factor in the susceptibility to infection. The only condition that seems to be enhanced by iron supplementation is malaria, probably due to the pathogenesis of this disease. Nevertheless, data in this regard are far from conclusive.

EFFECT OF IRON-FORTIFIED FOODS ON INFECTION DURING INFANCY

Three field studies testing the effect of iron-fortified foods on infection during infancy have been carried out in Chile. The Chilean government sponsors a supplemental food program, the National Supplementary Food Programme (NSFP), that provides free milk to children. The program has considerable prestige and acceptance. It provides 3 kg of full-fat milk per month for infants 0 to 6 months of age, then 2 kg for infants up to 24 months of age, and it reaches more than 80% of Chilean children. The milk provided by the NSFP is not iron-fortified. The children enrolled in these field studies were of middle to low socioeconomic status, living in houses built of solid material, with running water, a sewage system, and electricity.

Study 1

The study population lived in Santiago, Chile in an area served by two outpatient clinics of the National Health System (NHS). Infants for this study were selected randomly from participants in a larger field trial designed to determine the effects of iron-fortified milk on the iron nutritional status of infants (39). The larger field trial prospectively followed infants who had received two types of milk from 3 to 15 months of age. The infants were randomly assigned to an iron-fortified milk group ($n = 198$) or a non-iron-fortified group ($n = 184$). The iron-fortified milk group received a full fat (26%) powdered milk fortified with 15 mg of iron as ferrous sulfate, 100 mg of ascorbic acid, 1,500 IU of vitamin A, and 400 IU of vitamin D per 100 g of powder. The iron-fortified product was slightly acidified (total acidity = 2.5 g lactic acid/L) in order to discourage its consumption by other members of the family. The non-iron-fortified milk was a nonacidified similar powdered product. Both milks were provided through the clinic, and there was no noticeable difference in milk consumption between groups. Solid foods were introduced to all infants according to the usual practice in Chile: fruits and juices at 2 months, vegetables and meats at 4 months, legumes at 6 months, and table foods at 9 months of age.

Partially or fully weaned 3-month-old infants were considered for inclusion in the morbidity study if they met the following criteria: birth weight > 2,500 g, and free of perinatal illness, chronic disease, malnutrition, blood transfusion, or iron therapy. Seventy-four recipients of iron-fortified milk and 76 control infants were enrolled in the study (40).

Both groups received home visits by a trained field nurse every week, and mothers were instructed to keep a daily record of symptoms and signs. A standardized form was provided to record the following: number and character of the stools (formed, pasty, liquid, mucus, or blood), cough and/or wheezing with or without fever, and nasal discharge. One episode of diarrhea was defined as the presence of liquid stools for more than 24 hr. One episode of respiratory illness was defined as cough and/or wheezing for a duration of at least 5 days. Second episodes were those occurring after 7 or more symptom-free days. Every 2 weeks, the nurse obtained information on the infant's food intake. Consumption of iron-fortified milk was confirmed by serial determinations of iron in stools.

Infants at 3, 9, and 15 months of age were seen at the clinic, where anthropometric measurements and determinations of iron nutritional status were performed. Blood sampling was delayed for those children who were clinically ill at the time of a scheduled clinic visit.

Criteria for exclusion from the study were (a) hemoglobin levels below 9 g/dl at 9 months of age; (b) failure to follow the protocol; (c) less than 45 completed morbidity forms: (d) less than the level of iron in stools previously determined as proof of consistent iron-fortified milk intake; and (e) breast-feeding exclusively for more than 120 days. Fifty cases were not evaluated due to prolonged breast-feeding. Thus, the data from 53 infants receiving iron-fortified milk and 47 receiving non-iron-fortified milk were analyzed.

The prevalence of anemia and iron deficiency was significantly less in the iron-fortified group at 9 or 12 months of age. There were no differences between the two groups in the percentage of undernourished infants. No subjects were below 75% of the 50th percentile of NCHS standards for weight for age. The socioeconomic conditions of the two groups were similar.

The mean number of episodes of diarrhea was 1.1 per year per child in the iron-fortified group and 1.2 per year per child in the non-iron-fortified group. The figure for lower respiratory infections was 3.9 per year per child in both groups. In the iron-fortified group, 49.1% of infants and, in the non-iron-fortified group, 38.3% never developed diarrhea. The incidence of respiratory infection was 5.7% and 10.6% for the iron-fortified and non-iron-fortified groups, respectively. All differences were not statistically significant.

The main result of this prospective controlled study was to demonstrate that iron supplementation of milk at doses sufficient to eradicate iron deficiency anemia did not result in a significantly increased incidence of diarrheal or respiratory illness.

Study 2

This regional field trial was conducted to determine if the results of the first study could be reproduced under the standard operating conditions of the NHS clinics. The premise was that replacement of the non-iron-fortified formula distributed by the NHS with the iron-fortified formula would prevent iron deficiency in the vast majority of Chilean children reached through this program.

Two groups of spontaneously weaned infants were studied between June 1978 and February 1980 in all of the NHS clinics in the central area of Santiago. Infants born before July 31, 1978 continued on the regular non-iron-fortified milk program, which consisted of 3 kg of full-fat powdered milk per month until the age of 6 months, and 2 kg/month thereafter. Infants born after August 1, 1978, were given an equivalent amount of acidified iron-fortified milk with ascorbic acid as the control group. Health care was identical for the two groups. Detailed medical and nutritional status information was collected for 585 infants born in June and July who received non-iron-fortified milk and 654 infants born in August and September who received iron-fortified milk. These infants were followed until at least 9 months of age.

At 9 and 15 months of age, laboratory tests of iron nutritional status were performed on a subsample of approximately 200 infants in each group. These subsamples were randomly selected from the infants being followed in the seven participating clinics. Infants were selected on the basis of whether they were actually consuming the prescribed milk without consideration for other demographic factors such as birth weight. Clinic personnel provided well-baby care, took anthropometric measurements, and treated illnesses.

Initially, the general characteristics of the two groups were similar. There were no differences in birth weight, socioeconomic condition, maternal age, or parity. Breast feeding was actively encouraged at the clinics. The data on exclusive breast feeding were comparable for both groups, indicating that the introduction of the iron-fortified formula had no effect on duration of breast feeding. The percentage of infants born in August and September who actually consumed the acidified milk, excluding those who were breast-fed, varied between 70% and 80% from 3 to 15 months of age. Mothers who stated that their infants rejected the acidified milk were allowed to switch to the regular milk. It was very difficult to determine whether it was the infant or the mother who rejected the acidified milk.

There was a highly significant difference ($p < 0.001$) in all laboratory parameters of iron nutritional status between the two groups measured at 9 and 15 months of age. The percentage of iron-deficient subjects was lower in the iron-fortified group. The incidence of anemia in the iron-fortified group was 11.8% at 9 months and 5.5% at 15 months of age compared to 32.5% at 9 months and 29.9% at 15 months of age in the control group. At 15 months of age, only 3.8% of the infants who took iron-fortified milk for more than 10 months were anemic compared to 12.5% of those taking the iron-fortified milk for less than 10 months.

During the summer months of the southern hemisphere (November through February), when diarrhea tends to be prevalent, the group receiving iron-fortified milk had a lower incidence of diarrhea than the group receiving non-iron-fortified milk. The differences between the groups were statistically significant for the months of November and February. No group differences in the incidence of diarrhea were observed during the winter months. Moreover, there were no seasonal differences in the incidence of respiratory infections between the two groups.

In summary, the regional field trial confirmed the positive effect of the well-tolerated acidified, iron-fortified milk on the iron nutritional status of infants. There also appeared to be a positive effect of iron fortification on growth, particularly in low-birth-weight infants. This effect may have been due, in part, to less sharing of the acidified, iron-fortified milk within the family. In addition, the acidified, iron-fortified milk seemed to offer some protection against diarrhea in the summer months. However, the effect of the iron could not be separated from the effect of acidification.

Study 3

This study evolved from our most recently completed field trial of iron-fortified foods. In this study, infants who were being breast-fed adequately at 3 months of age were randomly assigned to one of two groups: either a group receiving heme iron-fortified rice cereal as a weaning food at 4 months of age and continuing through 12 months of age; or a group receiving the common solid foods that caregivers of Chilean infants are instructed to use (a meat–cereal–vegetable soup, fruits, and fruit juices at 4 months, legumes at 6 months, and table foods at 9 months of age). Infants who were obtaining > 50% of their expected energy intake from sources other than human milk were assigned either to a group receiving non-acidified fortified milk with 15 mg of elemental iron as ferrous sulfate per liter of reconstituted milk plus 100 mg of ascorbic acid, or to a group receiving regular non-iron-fortified milk provided by the NHS. Each group consisted originally of approximately 100 infants.

All infants enrolled in the study were full term and essentially healthy. They were seen monthly at the clinic for checkups, anticipatory guidance, and anthropometry, and they could come to the clinic whenever they were ill. Each home was visited weekly by a field nurse who completed a dietary survey and morbidity questionnaire similar to that used in Study 1.

Growth and development were similar in all groups. Breast-fed infants tended to be heavier during the first 6 to 9 months of age, but their weights were at the 50th percentile of the NCHS by 1 year of age. Deficient iron nutritional status, as measured by low iron stores and anemia, decreased in incidence across groups as follows: the non-iron-fortified early weaned infants, unfortified breast-fed infants, iron-fortified breast-fed infants, and fortified milk-fed infants.

These results illustrate the partial protection offered infants by breast feeding and the effectiveness of feeding an iron-fortified product consumed consistently from 3 to 4 months of age.

The incidence of mild diarrhea (less than 1 day's duration), diarrhea of more than 1 day's duration, and upper respiratory or lower respiratory disease was identical in all groups (Fig. 1). Otitis media was also uncommon. Seasonal variation showed its usual influence on prevalence of diarrheal and respiratory disease, without affecting any particular set of infants (Fig. 2).

Tunnesen and Oski (41) have recently reported on the effects of feeding whole cow's milk versus iron-fortified formula to infants after 6 months of age. At 12 months of age, the 69 infants receiving cow's milk had evidence of a lower iron status as measured by serum ferritin, erythrocyte protoporphyrin, and mean corpuscular volume and an increased incidence of anemia, as compared to 98 infants receiving iron-fortified formula. There was no evidence of untoward effects. The incidence of otitis media, wheezing, nasal discharge or congestion, diaper rash, constipation or guaiac-positive stools, or hospital admissions did not differ. Diarrhea, however, was more frequent in the infants fed cow's milk. A bias in this study may be the parental decision to give cow's milk instead of an infant formula when both were provided free of charge.

In conclusion, in places where sanitation and disadvantaged living conditions markedly increase the susceptibility to infection, at least one study seemed to demonstrate that large doses of oral iron for adults and parenteral iron for 2-month-old infants moderately increased the incidence of certain

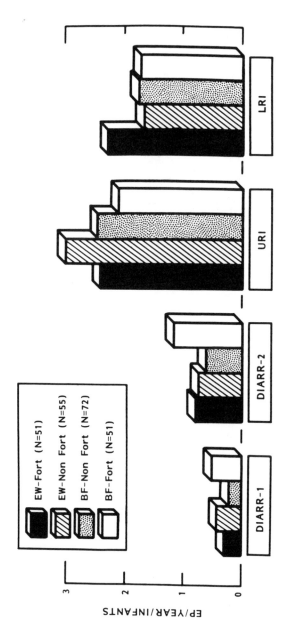

FIG. 1. Incidence of diarrhea in early weaned (EW) or breast-fed (BF), fortified (fort), or nonfortified (nonfort) infants from Study 3. Mild diarrhea of less than 1 day in duration (DIARR-1), moderate diarrhea (DIARR-2), upper respiratory infection (URI), and lower respiratory infection (LRI).

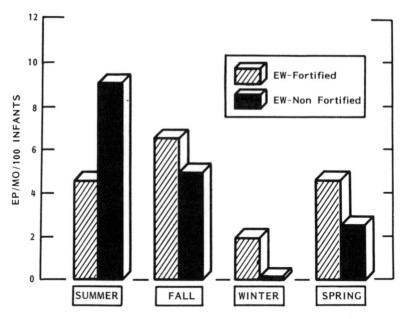

FIG. 2. Incidence of mild, moderate, or severe diarrhea for infants in Study 3 according to seasons (Summer, Fall, Winter, and Spring) recorded in clinic visits.

illnesses, particularly malaria. However, in all of these subjects, because multiple nutritional deficiencies were not adequately controlled, these effects could not be attributed exclusively to iron. Therefore, under usual circumstances in most areas of the world, oral iron therapy is not associated with increased rates of infection. More research is needed in the use of parenteral iron preparations in infancy, particularly in regions where there is a high prevalence of malaria. All current evidence indicates that iron fortification of foods is not associated with increased susceptibility to infection; moreover, there is some evidence that an adequate iron nutritional status may be beneficial.

REFERENCES

1. Thelander, L., Fraslund, A., and Thelander, M. (1983): Continual presence of oxygen and iron required for mammalian ribonucleotide reduction: possible regulation mechanism. *Biochem. Biophys. Res. Commun.*, 110:859–865.
2. Reichard, P., and Ehrenberg, A. (1983): Ribonucleotide reductase—a radical enzyme. *Science,* 221:514–519.
3. Joynson, D. H. M., Jacobs, A., Walker, D. M., and Dolby, A. E. (1972): Defect of cell-mediated immunity in patients with iron-deficiency anaemia. *Lancet,* 2:1058.

4. Vyas, D., and Chandra, R. K. (1984): Functional implications of iron deficiency. In: *Iron Nutrition in Infancy and Childhood,* edited by A. Stekel. Raven Press: New York, p. 45.
5. Chandra, R. K., and Saraya, A. K. (1975): Impaired immunocompetence associated with iron deficiency. *J. Pediatr.,* 86:899.
6. Macdougall, L. G., Anderson, R., McNab, G. M., and Katz, J. (1975): The immune response in iron-deficient children: impaired cellular defense mechanisms with altered humoral components. *J. Pediatr.,* 86:833.
7. Krantman, H. J., Young, S. R., O'Donnell, C. M., Rachelefsky, G. S., and Stiehm, E. R. (1982): Immune function in pure iron deficiency. *Am. J. Dis. Child.,* 136:840.
8. Chandra, R. K. (1975): Impaired immunocompetence associated with iron deficiency. *J. Pediatr.,* 86:899–902.
9. Bhaskaram, C., and Reddy, V. (1975): Cell-mediated immunity in iron and vitamin-deficient children. *Br. Med. J.,* 3:522.
10. Kulapongs, P., Vithayasai, V., Suskind, R., and Olson, R. E. (1974): Cell-mediated immunity and phagocytosis and killing function in children with severe iron-deficiency anaemia. *Lancet,* 2:689–91.
11. Chandra, R. K. (1973): Reduced bactericidal capacity of polymorphs in iron deficiency. *Arch. Dis. Child.,* 48:864–866.
12. Yetgin, S., Altay, C., Ciliv, G., and Laleli, Y. (1979): Myeloperoxidase activity and bactericidal function of PMN in iron deficiency. *Acta Haematol.,* 61:10–14.
13. Moore, L. L., and Humbert, J. R. (1984): Neutrophil bactericidal dysfunction towards oxidant radical-sensitive microorganisms during experimental iron deficiency. *Pediatr. Res.,* 18:684–689.
14. Babior, B. M. (1983): The respiratory burst of phagocytes. *J. Clin. Invest.,* 73:599–601.
15. Ambruso, D. R., and Johnston, R. B., Jr. (1981): Lactoferrin enhances hydroxyl radical production by human neutrophils, neutrophil particulate fractions, and an enzymatic generating system. *J. Clin. Invest.,* 67:352–60.
16. Walter, T., Arredondo, S., Arevalo, N., and Stekel, A. (1986): Effect of iron therapy on phagocytosis and bactericidal activity in neutrophils of iron-deficient infants. *Am. J. Clin. Nutr.,* 44:877–882.
17. Murakawa, H., Bland, C. E., Willis, W. T., and Dallman, P. R. (1987): Iron deficiency and neutrophil function: different rates of correction of the depressions in oxidative burst and myeloperoxidase activity after iron treatment. *Blood,* 69:1464–1468.
18. Weinberg, E. (1978): Iron and infection. *Microbiol. Rev.,* 42:45–66.
19. Olivares, M., Walter, T., Osorio, M., Chadud, P., and Schlesinger, L. (1989): The anemia of a mild viral infection: the measles vaccine as a model. *Pediatrics* (scheduled for publication).
20. Trousseau, A. (1882): *Lectures on clinical medicine.* New Sydeham Society, London.
21. McFarlane, H., Reddy, S., Adcock, K. J., Adeshina, H., Cooke, A. R., and Akene, J. (1970): Immunity transferrin and survival in kwashiorkor. *Br. Med. J.,* 4:268–270.
22. McFarlane, H., Okubadejo, M., and Reddy, S. (1972): Transferrin and *Staphylococcus aureus* in kwashiorkor. *Am. J. Clin. Pathol.,* 57:587–591.
23. Murray, M. J., Murray, A. B., Murray, C. J., and Murray, M. B. (1975): Refeeding—malaria and hyperferraemia. *Lancet,* 1:653–654.
24. Murray, M. J., and Murray, A. B. (1975): Starvation suppression and refeeding activation of infection. An ecological necessity? *Lancet,* 1:123–125.
25. Murray, M. J., Murray, A. B., Murray, M. B., and Murray, C. J. (1978): The adverse effect of iron repletion on the course of certain infections. *Br. Med. J.,* 1:113–115.
26. Mackay, H. N. M. (1928): Anaemia in infancy: its prevalence and prevention. *Arch. Dis. Child.,* 3:117–146.
27. Andelman, M. B., and Sered, B. R. (1966): Utilization of dietary iron by term infants. *Arch. Dis. Child.,* 111:45–55.
28. Burman, D. (1972): Hemoglobin levels in normal infants aged 3 to 24 months, and the effect of iron. *Arch. Dis. Child.,* 47:261.
29. Lovric, V. A. (1970): Normal haematologic values in children aged 6 to 36 months and sociomedical implications. *Med. J. Aust.,* 2:366–377.
30. Cantwell, R. J. (1972): Iron deficiency anaemia of infancy. *Clin. Pediatr.,* 11:403–449.
31. Valassi-Adam, H., Nassika, E., Kattamis, C., and Matsaniotis, N. (1976): Immunoglobulin levels in children with homozygous beta-thalassemia. *Acta Paediatr. Scand.,* 165:145–155.
32. Barry, D. M. J., and Reeve, A. W. (1974): Iron and infection in the newborn. *Lancet,* 2:1385.

33. Narlon, A., Gentry, L., and Merigan, T. C. (1971): Septicemia and *Pasteurella pseudotuberculosis* and liver disease. *Arch. Intern. Med.,* 127:947–949.
34. Oppenheimer, S. J., MacFarlane, S. B. J., Moody, J. B., Bunari, O., and Hendrickage, R. G. (1986): Effect of iron prophylaxis on morbidity due to infectious disease. *Trans. R. Soc. Trop. Med. Hyg.,* 80:596–602.
35. Barry, D. M. J., and Reeve, A. W. (1977): Increased incidence gram-negative neonatal sepsis with intramuscular iron administration. *Pediatrics,* 60:908–912.
36. Leikin, S. L. (1960): The use of intramuscular iron in the prophylaxis of the iron deficiency anemia of prematurity. *Am. J. Dis. Child.,* 99:739–745.
37. Salmi, T., Hanninen, P., and Peltonen, T. (1963): Applicability of chelated iron in the care of prematures. *Acta Paediatr. Scand.,* 140:114–115.
38. Oppenheimer, S. J., Gibson, F. D., McFarlane, S. B., et al. (1986): Iron supplementation increases prevalence and effects of malaria: report on clinical studies in Papua New Guinea. *Trans. R. Soc. Trop. Med. Hyg.,* 80:603–612.
39. Stekel, A., Olivares, M., Cayazzo, M., Chadud, P., Llaguno, S., and Pizarro, F. (1988): Prevention of iron deficiency by milk fortification. II: A field trial with a full fat acidified milk. *Am. J. Clin. Nutr.,* 47:265–269.
40. Heresi, G., Olivares, M., Pizarro, F., Cayazzo, M., and Stekel, A. (1987): Effect of an iron fortified milk on morbidity in infancy: a field trial. *Nutr. Res.,* 7:915–922.
41. Tunnessen, W. W., and Oski, F. A. (1987): Consequences of starting whole cow milk at 6 months of age. *J. Pediatr.,* 111:813–816.

Dietary Iron: Birth to Two Years,
edited by L. J. Filer, Jr.
Raven Press, Ltd., New York © 1989.

Discussion

Dr. Yip: You said that the infants in your study had no obvious increased rates of infection. Actually, you need a much larger population to show such a difference.

Dr. Walter: Yes, I realize that. However, it was clear that iron-deficient infants had impaired bactericidal function but did not become sicker. Of course, these infants were all well nourished otherwise.

Dr. Dallman: Isn't it true that if large numbers of malaria parasites are detected in the blood, they are in the most severe iron-deficient cases? I am very impressed with the Oppenheimer data that indicate that iron dextran injections do not make malaria worse.

Dr. Walter: I cannot interpret the malaria data.

Dr. Oski: Did Oppenheimer include serum iron values so that one could see if there were true differences between the two groups as a consequence of iron administration?

Dr. Walter: The anemia caused by the malaria was so overwhelming that the iron dextran did not make any difference in iron status at the end of the year. The point is that it is only in severely infected underprivileged populations in certain areas of the world where one probably has to be careful with added iron. Certainly, it is not a concern in more normal environments.

Dr. Oski: If one examines serum iron levels several days after an injection of iron dextran, the values are frightening. They are often around 1,000 µg/dl, which is almost what one would observe in iron poisoning. That is the time one would expect to observe an effect on infection, not 8 to 10 months later.

Dr. Walravens: Does iron have its effect through the production of more red blood cells, thereby facilitating an increase in number of malaria parasites?

Dr. Yip: It is because there are more young red blood cells. Malaria is actually in a different category of infection than other types of viral or bacterial infections in its association with iron deficiency or iron treatment. We understand the mechanism better. In those regions where malaria is endemic, the people who have the most active disease and the most parasitemia are those who have the highest reticulocyte counts. If one suddenly treats a person who has been severely iron-deficient, there will be a sudden increase in the synthesis of new red blood cells, which gives subclinical malaria a chance to flourish. Similarly, if the iron nutritional status of a group is much better at a given time, these persons are going to produce fewer young red blood cells. Therefore, if two groups are exposed equally to malaria, the iron-sufficient group will manifest a more severe spectrum of the disease. It is the number of young red blood cells that correlates well with iron status.

Dr. Walter: I guess the message is to prevent malaria.

Dr. Yip: Yes, that is correct.

Dr. Owen: In your comparisons of body weight against the NCHS charts, you observe what many people are finding, i.e., that there is an excess of weight for age in the period between 2 and 7 months, and then body weight tends to be closer to the standards. I believe this is an artifact of the chart.

Dr. Oski: Why do you say it is an artifact of the chart? If one compares breast-fed infants with non-breast-fed infants, there is a period of time when the breast-fed infants are very, very chubby, and then they become lean after about 1 year of age. We find that they don't retain that baby fat.

Dr. Owen: I think it is an artifact of the chart because the chart is based on formula-fed infants.

Dr. Oski: However, there is a difference between breast-fed and formula-fed infants.

Dr. Owen: Yes.

Dr. Walter: The length-for-age curves do exactly the same thing. These curves are fine until about 6 to 7 months of age and then they fall off, more markedly in male than in female infants. We would like to determine whether zinc has anything to do with this because it is similar to what Dr. Walravens reported.

Dr. Yip: During the last 6 months, I have been heavily involved in the evaluation of the reference curves for growth in terms of how the original samples were obtained and how the curves were constructed. We are fairly well convinced that somewhere between 9 and 24 months, the current reference values for length-for-age are significantly higher than they should be. Also, there is a problem with the growth data somewhere between 36 and 60 months. This is because the reference material was from the Fels Institute, and these children are taller and leaner for some reason than American children as a whole. If a national representative sample of infants and children is plotted on the current chart, we observe what you do. We are contemplating whether we want to release a revision of the standard growth chart.

Dr. Filer: The incidence of obesity among children will be distorted if you revise the charts.

Dr. Yip: Also, the method of measurement changes at 24 months. Therefore, there are several major problems. It is very difficult, especially for research purposes, to compare growth status from one age group to another.

Dr. Walter: There are a lot of problems with the charts, but nevertheless we have very low serum zinc levels in these children. We did follow the recommendations regarding time of day and fasting, and the samples were measured by a good laboratory. Thus, I believe that the techniques are valid.

Dr. Walravens: Due to diurnal variation in serum zinc levels, it is important to collect blood at about the same time of day.

Dr. Owen: In your study, the unfortified milk group had an incidence of anemia of 27%. What age were these infants?

Dr. Walter: They were 12 months of age.

Dr. Walravens: Did you say that the cereal was heme-fortified in the study of breast-fed infants?

Dr. Walter: Yes. It contained 5% bovine hemoglobin.

Dr. Oski: What is the overall incidence of smoking in the parents of your infant population?

Dr. Walter: It is very low.

Dr. Oski: A number of studies have shown that the incidence of diarrhea in infants fed cow's milk is lower than the incidence of diarrhea in infants fed formula. It has been postulated that the reason for the lowered incidence is the presence of an immunoglobulin in cow's milk that is not present in heat-treated formula.

Dr. Owen: It has also been suggested that part of the difference might relate to the presence of butterfat in the cow's milk in contrast to the formula, in which the fat is from vegetable sources.

Dr. Walter: Stool volume of cow's-milk-fed infants is more than two times greater than that of formula-fed infants. Thus, it is possible that many of the diarrheal episodes reported were actually large volumes of watery or mushy stools and not acute infectious diarrhea.

Dr. Oski: Except for otitis media, which was directly observed, all of these events of diarrhea were identified by history. I do not want to attach a lot of significance to such observations.

Dr. Filer: Some of the information that you presented shows that iron supplementation can either prevent infection or cause infection. As a summary, could you give some guidelines regarding the clinical or environmental conditions when it is appropriate to supplement with iron? Also, in those conditions in which iron might cause infection, would you want to provide any additional iron whatsoever? If iron is given, what form and dose level would you want to provide?

Dr. Walter: In all of our studies, the cow's milk was fortified with 15 mg of elemental iron as ferrous sulfate per liter. Thus, I am not talking about subtle amounts of iron. Where possible, infants worldwide should receive bioavailable iron during the first year of life. We and others have shown that this is best accomplished by food fortification, and the food of choice for fortification in infancy is milk. Milk for infants can be safely fortified with iron in any part of the world.

Dr. Filer: Even in tropical countries where malaria is rampant?

Dr. Walter: Yes. The evidence does not show that iron fortification of milk causes any problems with infection.

Dr. Owen: Would you comment on the level of iron fortification?

Dr. Walter: The level of iron to be added must be determined by field tests. One must be very knowledgeable about the iron content of the overall diet of the infant population in order to recommend a level. In countries where there are other sources of iron in the diet, lower levels of iron fortification may be adequate. However, in countries where there are no other sources of dietary iron during the first year of life, higher levels of fortification may be needed. I believe that the cutoff mark should be around 12 mg of elemental iron per liter of formula. In countries where there are other sources of iron, perhaps it should be at the 12 mg level or below, and in countries where there are no other sources of iron, perhaps it should be 12 mg/liter or more.

Dr. Dallman: I think that we need clinical studies on levels of iron fortification. Such studies would not be difficult to do in a country like Chile. Chile provides an ideal setting for checking whether 6 or 8 mg of iron per liter are equivalent and give the same physiological effect. One might want to consider the infection issue separately and consider the risk of enteric infections versus systemic infections. I think that the risk of iron in formula affecting systemic infections is low because the difference in transferrin saturation of infants who are being fed iron-fortified formula versus those being fed non-iron-fortified formula is only 3% to 5%.

When parenteral iron is given, however, transferrin becomes completely saturated and cannot perform its bacteriostatic function of keeping iron from bacteria that require it for growth. This is why there are more problems with this form of iron administration. We may find that we are wrong about the effects of oral iron on systemic infections; however, enteric infections may be another matter. I have heard the concern expressed that if one gives iron at the time of breast feeding, lactoferrin, which supposedly performs a similar function in the intestine as transferrin does in the blood, becomes saturated. I do not know whether this is true for formula. In cow's milk, transferrin, not lactoferrin, is the major iron-binding protein, and I am not sure whether one can saturate transferrin or not. The fact that Dr. Walter is showing us data that do not indicate a striking difference in enteric infections is reassuring.

Dr. Oski: I believe unequivocally that formula-fed infants all over the world should be provided with an iron-fortified formula during the first year of life. I know of no compelling evidence whatsoever that iron-fortified formulas increase the risk of systemic infections or gastrointestinal infections. I think that there are two issues that should be examined: first, the level of iron fortification (i.e., 6, 8, or 12 mg/liter) is worthy of examination to establish the lowest amount of added iron to achieve the desired clinical result; second, I think that someone should do some simple studies on the microflora of the gut to establish their relationship to iron in the diet.

Dr. Dallman: There is an exhaustive analysis from Holland of gut microflora of breast-fed, non-iron-fortified-formula-fed, and iron-fortified-formula-fed infants. Six milligrams per liter of iron resulted in major changes in the gut microflora within 1 week.

Dr. Oski: In our country, bacterial infections represent, at the most, 10% of the total infections in children; the rest are mainly viral.

Dr. Dallman: Yes, I think we can be fairly sure that iron fortification makes a big difference in intestinal microflora, but whether it makes a difference in health is another question.

Dr. Oski: Even the introduction of solid foods will change the gut microflora in breast-fed infants.

Dr. Filer: Should infants be switched to a low-iron formula when they have diarrhea or an infection?

Dr. Walter: We do not switch formula. There is no rationale for doing that.

Dr. Dallman: If we start recommending such a procedure, we will have the same thing happening as has happened with soy formulas, i.e., it will be too easy to use infection as a reason for formula switching.

Dr. Oski: There is no evidence for that recommendation.

Dr. Filer: The single most difficult problem identified by the practicing pediatrician is the perception that iron-fortified formulas cause constipation. Dr. Walter, you and Dr. Oski have stated that there are no differences in the stool patterns of infants fed iron-fortified formula or a non-iron-fortified formula. How do you deal with the myth that iron-fortified formula causes constipation?

Dr. Oski: I do not know how to deal with the myth. Thus, I would eliminate the problem by not offering the non-iron-fortified formula.

Dr. Walter: I cannot comment because our study was done with iron-fortified cow's milk, and there is a difference between this and formula.

Dr. Oski: There is not one shred of evidence, other than anecdotal reports from some parents, that constipation is associated with iron-fortified formulas. Carefully controlled studies in adults (which included placebos that had the proper color) have failed to show that there is an increased incidence of gastrointestinal symptoms when taking iron, even in large quantities.

Dr. Dallman: The best studies of the side effects of ferrous sulfate preparations were done in Gothenburg on about 3,000 blood donors given large doses of oral iron. However, 1-year-old infants are not good at complaining about gastrointestinal side effects.

Dr. Walter: In our studies of behavioral and cognitive development, we gave a group of 300 infants ferrous sulfate or placebo for 10 days. These children were seen by a nurse four times in 10 days. There was no difference between the groups in side effects during this time.

Dr. Dallman: I would like to comment on the statement that Dr. Oski made that all formulas should be iron-fortified, and formulas without added iron (or those with less than 3 mg/liter) should be eliminated. I certainly agree with that feeling in many respects, but I am leery of stating it that strongly. I think we have to remember that when we compare the amount of iron in human milk with that in formula, we have a bigger deviation than any other nutrient. We do not know a lot of things about iron nutrition. However, one can justify raising the iron level in formula considerably above the human milk level on the basis of bioavailability, and one can argue for four times as much as a minimum figure because bioavailability is that much less; but 12 mg of iron is considerably above that in human milk. Maybe there is some biological rationale for the iron content of human milk, something that we have not learned about yet or something that has to do with immune function that has not been recognized because not enough studies have been done. We always need to consider human milk as a starting point when deciding what to feed infants. I would feel better about making a definite statement if formulas had an iron level of 6 mg, which is not that much above 3 mg, but I am not as willing to go along with that position when the fortification level is 12 mg of iron.

Dr. Oski: What I said was that all milk should be iron-fortified. I also said that formula should be fortified with the least amount of iron that is effective.

Dr. Dallman: Until we know what that number is, I am content to have the unfortified formula available.

Dr. Oski: That least amount of iron required could be very easily measured. Early field trials with a formula providing 6 mg/liter of iron demonstrated that 6 mg was adequate.

Dr. Dallman: I suspect that an unstated reason so many pediatricians recommend and parents are still using a formula without added iron is that it is closer to human milk.

Dr. Oski: I do not think so at all.

Dr. Ziegler: I tend to agree with Dr. Dallman in that I have some uneasiness about phasing out non-iron-fortified formula. However, what use does it have? If you think that formula-fed infants should receive formulas with iron, who, then, should receive the nonfortified formula, other than those parents and pediatricians who resist use of the iron-fortified formula?

Dr. Dallman: One could argue that the non-iron-fortified formula is the formula of choice for the first 4 months of life of term infants because they do not need iron. I am not saying that one should recommend that, but I am saying that there may be no reasons for not doing that.

Dr. Filer: You need to remember that this approach would complicate the situation. In Andelman's study, infants who started on iron-fortified formula at the time of discharge from Cook County Hospital were compared with infants who were given iron-fortified formula upon their first clinic visit, which was 6 to 8 weeks of age in those days. These two groups had different hemoglobin distribution curves later in the first year of life, indicating that early iron administration was beneficial.

Dr. Dallman: My reservations are not based on any one study. I am saying that until we know the lowest level of iron that is effective in the majority of infants, I have reservations about making absolute statements against the use of low-iron formulas because they may turn out to have a place in infant feeding.

Dietary Iron: Birth to Two Years,
edited by L. J. Filer, Jr.
Raven Press, Ltd., New York © 1989.

Influence of Iron Nutrition on Work Capacity and Performance

Fernando E. Viteri

*Department of Nutritional Sciences, College of Natural Resources, University of
California, Berkeley, California 94720*

Interest in the effects of iron deficiency and anemia on physical work capacity and productivity has only recently developed (1). The key role of iron in the transport and utilization of oxygen explains the widely recognized fact that severely anemic individuals cannot carry out tasks involving muscular work. For this reason, it is amazing that individuals with 2 or 3 g/dl of hemoglobin (80–85% deficit) can continue to be physically active in regions where chronic iron deficiency is endemic. This phenomenon provides evidence for the known series of compensating mechanisms that come into play when iron deficiency develops slowly. In addition, limitations on spontaneous physical activity and overall "tiredness" are manifestations of chronic iron deficiency anemia only when the anemia is severe (hemoglobin level lower than 7 g/dl).

Iron deficiency is prevalent and particularly severe among tropical rural-poor populations that are dependent upon physically demanding tasks for survival and economic development. Such people are victims of chronic hunger, high rates of infection, and environmental deprivation that limit developmental stimuli and educational opportunities. Under these circumstances, it is difficult to isolate the effects of iron deficiency as a cause of "lack of ambition and general inactivity." In children, inadequate human milk feeding (primarily an urban phenomenon), poor weaning, generally inadequate feeding practices, and early repeated infections (including hookworm, whipworm, and malaria) are responsible for the high prevalence of anemia (2) (Table 1). These children are apathetic, listless, irritable, and have altered development and diminished growth velocity. These manifestations could easily be assigned to iron deficiency, overall malnutrition, lack of stimulation, chronic and/or repeated infections, or to several of these factors. At the same time, moderate and severe protein–energy malnutrition diminishes the severity of iron deficiency by slowing growth rates and, where loss of active tissue mass ensues, by a contraction of the total circulating hemoglobin mass (3,4).

141

TABLE 1. *Estimated prevalence of anemia in children by geographic region (1980)[a]*

Region	0–4 years		5–12 years	
	Percentage	Number[b]	Percentage	Number[b]
Africa	56	48.0	49	47.3
Latin America	26	13.7	26	18.1
East Asia[c]	20	3.2	22	5.6
South Asia	56	118.7	50	139.2
World[c]	43	193.5	37	217.4
Developed regions[d]	12	10.3	7	9.1
Developing regions	51	183.2	46	208.3

[a]From ref. 2.
[b]Numbers = millions.
[c]Excluding China.
[d]According to United Nations regions, including North America, Japan, Europe, Australia, New Zealand, and the Union of Soviet Socialist Republics.

TABLE 2. *Summary of studies in children exploring the effect of anemia and iron deficiency on physical work capacity.*

Population	Age (years)	Hemoglobin (g/dl)	Reference
Male/female	10–20	8.9–19.7	8

Main findings: Hemoglobin is directly associated with speed, strength, and sustained muscular effort; not so with the Harvard Step Test and Endurance Step Test (both near VO_2max).

Male/female	10–16	10.9–16.5	6

Main findings: Hemoglobin correlates with VO_2max but not when corrected for body weight or when groups of children by sex and age are studied independently.

Male/female	7–14	7.1–14.0	9

Main findings: Hemoglobin and body weight explain most variance in submaximal VO_2.

Male	12–15	Mean: 14.0 SD: 1.0	10

Main findings: Hemoglobin highly correlated with VO_2max. VO_2max also correlated with vitamin A and vitamin B_2 nutritional status.

Male/female	11–14.5	9.7–15.1	11

Main findings: Responses to iron and vitamins C, B, and B_2 were associated with decrements in submaximal VO_2. Changes in hemoglobin were negatively related to changes in VO_2 in standard submaximal work.

Male/female	4–7.5	2.9–11.5	5

Main findings: Five clinical cases; remarkable lack of correlation between hemoglobin and "exercise tolerance" in chronic anemia; not so in acute anemia; little improvement with transfusion.

Male/female	Mean: 14.0 SD: 2.3	Mean: 8.0 SD: 0.6	7

Main findings: VO_2 for a given work load was not affected by anemia. Heart rate was elevated and VO_2max reduced in anemic children even when expressed per kg of body weight or lean body mass.

The influence of iron deficiency on spontaneous physical activity of children has not been measured; and not many studies have explored the effect of anemia or iron deficiency on physical work capacity in children. Furthermore, results from such studies are far from clear (5–11). In general, mild to moderate anemia (hemoglobin concentration as low as 9.5 g/dl) fails consistently to affect submaximal oxygen uptake in school-age children (Table 2). Similarly, hemoglobin levels as low as 10.8 g/dl do not consistently reduce maximal aerobic power in 10- to 16-year-olds (6) (Fig. 1). These findings contrast with findings in the adult population, where consistently positive linear correlations are found between hemoglobin concentration and maximal work situations (12–14). It is possible that children may be able to compensate more efficiently for iron deficiency and anemia in terms of physical work capacity, that the methodology used to detect alterations in physical work performance in children is not as well standardized and precise as in adults, or both. The need for research in this area is evident.

Given the similarities in effects of iron deficiency on hematological and endocrine alterations in both adults and children, what is known from studies in the adult might be assumed to be relevant to infants and children until bet-

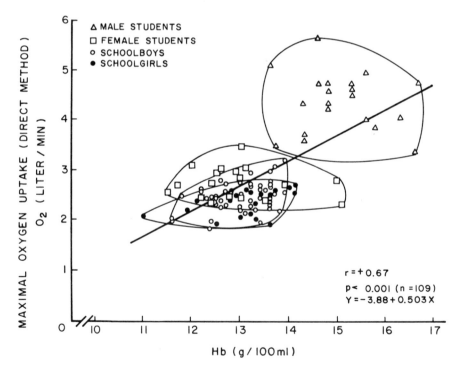

FIG. 1. Maximal aerobic capacity (VO2max) of children relative to hemoglobin concentration. (Reproduced from ref. 6 with permission from Alonquist & Wilmsell Periodical Co., © 1971.)

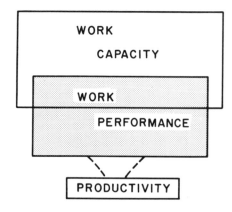

FIG. 2. Schematic model of an approach to the study of productivity.

ter definitions of specific compensatory mechanisms are developed. Similarly, the mechanisms by which iron deficiency impairs physical working capacity and performance in severely iron-deficient animal models may serve as a guide for additional research on the effects of iron deficiency on physical activity and performance in humans (adults and children).

The relationship between work capacity, work performance, and productivity is the result of complex processes (Fig. 2), with overlap between the conditions that determine each component (Figs. 3 and 4).

Briefly, the genetic makeup of the individual (host) and interaction with the environment and various agents (some nutrients) determine the growth, health, and nutritional status of the individual (Fig. 3). Human development, in turn, is determined by the final functional expression of these components at the point

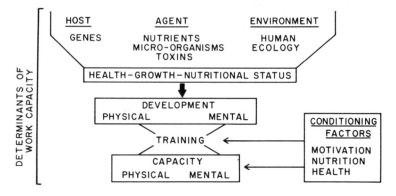

FIG. 3. Diagram of factors that affect work capacity.

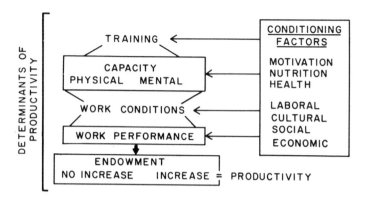

FIG. 4. Diagram of factors that affect work performance and productivity.

where they interact. The addition of a purposeful component, identified as training (including education), provides the final specific modulation to the level of general development, expressed as capacity to perform specific tasks.

Figure 4 illustrates the determinants of a specific performance of work. Here, additional and more specific training as well as the development of greater dexterity in a specific task can improve performance, building upon an already existing capacity. The conditions under which this capacity is to be exercised as productive work as well as the social and economic meaning of such work also determine performance. The final factor is the value of such performance in modification of human endowment. A positive modification may not necessarily imply an improvement in economic terms. For example, more satisfying or edifying expenditure of leisure time constitutes a positive modification of human endowment, particularly in children, and, as such, must be considered a productive human performance.

THE ROLE OF IRON IN THE DEVELOPMENT OF PHYSICAL WORK CAPACITY

Body Size and Composition, Health, and General Nutrition

Physical work capacity, expressed as work performed per unit time, is positively correlated to body size, lean body mass, and, more specifically, to the absolute amount of active tissue mass, of which functional muscle mass is the largest component (15–17). In controlled animal experiments, iron deficiency has consistently demonstrated a negative effect on growth that is reversible when the deficiency is corrected (18). A plausible explanation for this phenomenon is reduced food intake, which is exacerbated by decreased feed efficiency in deficient animals. This effect appears to occur only when the dietary-induced deficiency is moderate to severe (19,20). In human populations in developing countries who show both inadequate growth and iron deficiency, the relative role of the iron deficit cannot be defined. However, a basis exists for implicating iron deficiency as contributing to poor growth, poor muscle mass development, poor health, and poor general nutrition in such populations.

In the same ecological setting, iron-deficient children show growth deficits relative to non-iron-deficient children (21). Iron deficiency and poor growth may be the consequence of various phenomena that coincide in these children and serve as covariates.

Several immunological defects have been documented in iron-deficient humans and animals (22–24), which in the presence of infection may have a role in the magnitude of the "disease phenomenon" of developing populations. Indirect evidence (25) suggests that repeated infection hampers growth, food intake, iron absorption, and iron metabolism (26–29). Finally, iron deficiency has been associated with aberrations in eating patterns (pica, for example) that can increase the potential for infection with all of its consequences.

Iron-deficient animals have a reduced functional muscle mass (30) and iron-deficient anemic adults have a lower body mass index than non-iron-deficient individuals (31). Unfortunately, it is impossible to determine if this last finding is due to lower adiposity or to lower lean body (and muscle) mass, or if it occurs independent of iron deficiency. However, the fact that anemic iron-deficient adults react with higher oxygen consumption to cold exposure than their normal counterparts (31) suggests an additional mechanism by which iron deficiency may burden already marginally nourished, often-infected populations.

General Development

The capacity to perform work depends not only on the physical attributes of the individual but also on his/her cognitive and emotional development (32). Hormonal derangements demonstrated in iron-deficient humans (31,33,34) and animals (35–37) can also interfere with normal development, in particular alterations in thyroxine metabolism (36,37). Several enzymatic defects in the neuroendocrine axis and in the liver are other factors by which iron deficiency may interfere at critical stages of development (38,39).

Also important to development is the diminution in spontaneous activity demonstrated by iron-deficient rats relative to iron-sufficient controls (19,40) (Fig. 5) and by human adult groups in Sri Lanka (41) (Fig. 6). Diminished physical activity may be another mechanism involved in impaired growth (42).

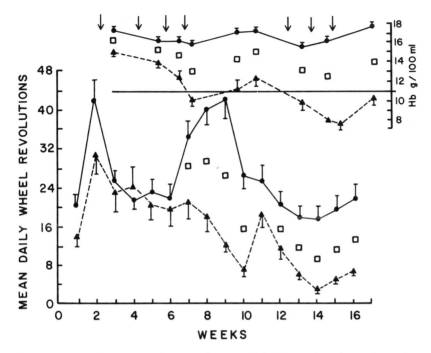

FIG. 5. Hemoglobin concentration and voluntary activity in anemic and control rats. Arrows indicate days when blood was drawn. Upper graph: mean ± SEM of concentration in control (——) and anemic rats (- -). Lower graph: mean ± SEM of spontaneous activity in the same rats. □ = $p < 0.05$. Taken from ref. 40.

Training

Until recently, nothing was known about the effect of iron deficiency on physical training or the converse effect of physical training on iron deficiency. Studies in growing (43–46) and in adult rats (47) have shown that physical training in iron-deficient rats is associated with a relative improvement in iron status compared to untrained, iron-deficient controls. Enhancement of iron absorption as a consequence of intense physical activity may be responsible for this improvement (47), together with mobilization of small amounts of storage iron toward the heart and other active muscles (43,44). However, very strict control of iron contamination of the training treadmill used in these studies markedly diminished differences in hemoglobin concentration and in iron-containing mitochondrial enzymes in muscle (46).

Although mild to moderate training improved endurance work significantly in both iron-deficient and iron-sufficient rats, the latter exhibited a greater response, indicating that iron deficiency limits the response to training. Maximal aerobic capacity (VO$_2$max) exhibits a small, often insignifi-

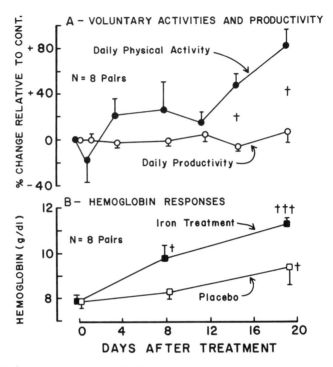

FIG. 6. Effect of iron treatment. **(A)** Changes in physical activity and productivity in eight pairs of female tea pickers in response to oral iron therapy (mean % ± SEM of control values). **(B)** Hemoglobin concentration of treated workers and placebo controls. $\dagger p < 0.05$; $\dagger\dagger\dagger p < 0.001$. (Reproduced from ref. 41 with permission from the *British Medical Journal*, © 1979.)

cant response to mild or moderate training independent of iron status. Consistently, trained and untrained anemic rats demonstrated significantly impaired performance in both endurance and maximal work when compared to normal controls (45) (Fig. 7).

No specific studies have been carried out to explore the effect of training in iron-deficient and control human subjects. In a double-blind study in Guatemala, 44 physically active adult agricultural workers (both anemic due to iron deficiency and nonanemic) were divided into two paired groups: one received therapeutic doses of iron, and the other received an identical placebo (48). Neither the subjects performing the Harvard Step Test (HST) nor the investigators knew which subject belonged to which group. The HST was performed at baseline and at 2-, 4-, and 16-week intervals. Although the treated subjects improved in hemoglobin concentration and hematocrit and HST, the placebo group did not change, suggesting that there was no training effect in this group (48). Similarly, 10 Ceylonese anemic individuals who received placebo for 16 days and performed maximum work tests every 4 days did not exhibit any training effect (14). Two drawbacks to the inter-

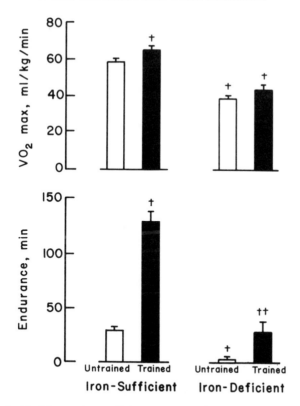

FIG. 7. Effect of training on iron-sufficient and iron-deficient rat VO_2max and endurance (mean ± SEM). $^+p < 0.05$ within training group. $^*p < 0.05$ between trained and untrained rats within a diet group. $^{++}p < 0.05$ between iron-deficient and iron-sufficient rats within a training group. (Reproduced from ref. 45 with permission from the American Physiological Society, © 1985.)

pretation of these results are apparent: (a) the training was far from intensive, and (b) Guatemalan subjects were already in good physical condition from living in the mountains.

MECHANISMS INVOLVED IN THE RELATIONSHIP BETWEEN IRON NUTRITION AND PHYSICAL WORK CAPACITY

Overall Physical Work Capacity

In humans, a linear relationship exists between hemoglobin concentration and the level of maximal work capacity by the HST (13,49) (Fig. 8) or by measurement of maximal aerobic capacity (VO_2max) (12,14,50,51). The

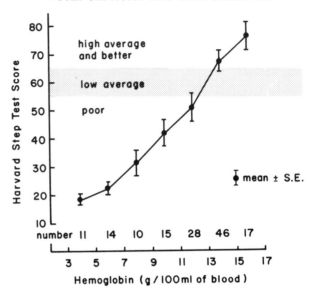

FIG. 8. Relationship between severe physical exercise performance, as measured by the Harvard Step Test score, and hemoglobin concentration in adult men. (Reproduced from ref. 13 with permission from W. B. Saunders, UK, © 1974.)

detailed studies of Gardner et al. (50) on female workers in Sri Lanka provided information on heart rate and lactic acid levels in response to standard exercise loads, all indicative of progressive limitations on heavy physical work in direct relation to the deficit in hemoglobin concentration (severity of anemia). Similar results were reported by Celsing and Ekblom (52). At the same blood lactate concentration, anemic subjects were closer to their VO_2max than these same subjects to their respective VO_2max when the anemia was corrected. VO_2max increased parallel to hemoglobin concentration. At a lactate concentration of 4 mM, VO_2 in the corrected state or before anemia was induced was higher than VO_2max when moderate anemia (Hgb = 11 ± 0.8 g/dl) had been induced by bleeding. These findings suggest that the reduction of VO_2max in anemia is more limiting than lactate accumulation.

Similar results have been obtained with rats under rigorously standardized conditions (18,40,53–55). Studies in iron-deficient rats (56,57) indicated that VO_2max decreased in relation to the decline in hemoglobin concentration with two different slopes. When hemoglobin levels were lower than 8 g/dl, the slope was steep, but when hemoglobin levels exceeded 9 g/dl in response to treatment, the slope was flat. The response in rats contrasts with data on humans that show no difference in slope whether hemoglobin levels decrease or whether they increase in response to iron therapy or transfusion (13,14,51).

Adaptation Mechanisms

Because oxygen delivery and utilization by active tissues are essential in order to maintain function, adaptation mechanisms compensate for the diminution in oxygen-carrying capacity induced by chronic iron deficiency anemia. Important among these mechanisms at rest and at submaximal exercise levels are well-documented elevations in cardiac output, the lowering of peripheral resistance with redirection of blood flow, and shift in the oxygen dissociation curve of hemoglobin towards maximizing oxygen delivery at low oxygen tensions (58–61). The elevation in cardiac output occurs through an increase in heart rate for a given exercise load, while oxygen extraction in the peripheral tissues also increases. Each mechanism contributes about 50% to the physiological adaptation when anemia is mild to moderate, i.e., a hemoglobin concentration > 9 g/dl (62). Among individuals with similar active tissue mass, maximal aerobic power, as defined by VO_2max, is dependent on circulating hemoglobin levels, since cardiac output does not increase significantly above normal in anemic states. On the contrary, a mild or nonsignificant reduction in VO_2max of 5% to 8% with hemoglobin levels around 11 to 12 g/dl is not unusual in otherwise healthy men (51,61). VO_2max, however, can be increased by hypertransfusion and by an adequate exercise training regimen among healthy individuals. In the first instance, an average of 18.9 $\pm$ 6.4 (SD) ml/min/g of change in hemoglobin/liter of blood has been documented (maximum Hgb near 20 g/dl). In the second instance, VO_2max can be increased by 20% or more (51,58). All of these mechanisms may compensate for the modest reduction in oxygen-carrying capacity that results from chronic moderate anemia in order to maintain adequate tissue oxygenation. However, when maximal or near-maximal aerobic capability is demanded, or when hemoglobin levels are so low (< 7 g/dl) as to compromise tissue oxygenation even with minimal effort, these compensatory mechanisms fail.

Several studies (63–66) have demonstrated enzymatic and composition changes in muscle at the cellular level in iron deficiency and the response to iron therapy. Substantial evidence indicates that iron deficiency occurs in twice as many individuals as those exhibiting anemia (67), since the latter condition is a relatively late manifestation of iron deficiency.

In the mid-1970s, a series of elegant functional studies examined the role of iron deficiency at the muscle level independent of anemia. They demonstrated that muscle function in the rat was impaired by iron deficiency, even when the capacity of the blood to deliver oxygen to muscle was still adequate. This impairment was caused by a series of structural and enzymatic deficiencies that reduced the oxidative capacity of muscle primarily by means of a decreased functional mitochondrial mass. Muscle capacity was probably further impaired by a lower intramuscular oxygen diffusion capacity consequent to a reduction in myoglobin. These defects resulted primarily in reduced endurance and submaximal work performance.

In growing rats, the sequence of changes in muscle as iron deficit progresses (Fig. 9) clearly shows a rapid decline in cytochrome c and transferrin saturation with progressive iron deficiency, followed shortly by a reduction in hemoglobin and myoglobin concentrations. All of these changes occur when liver iron reserves are exhausted (68). In iron-deficient adult rats, however, myoglobin reduction does not occur (69). Iron deficiency also produces substantial declines in the activity of key iron–sulfur proteins, mitochondrial oxidative enzymes, dehydrogenases, cytochromes, and flavoproteins involved in electron transport and oxidative phosphorylation. These changes reduce the mitochondrial capacity to produce high-energy phosphates (ATP) (30,70,71) and reduce markedly the bioenergetic function of mitochondria. Mitochondrial mass also appears to be reduced in muscle from iron-deficient rats (30). These alterations are further complicated in iron deficiency by the demonstrated decline in the α-glycerophosphate oxidase system that drives the operation of the α-glycerophosphate shuttle. This system, together with the malate–aspartate shuttle, contributes not only to

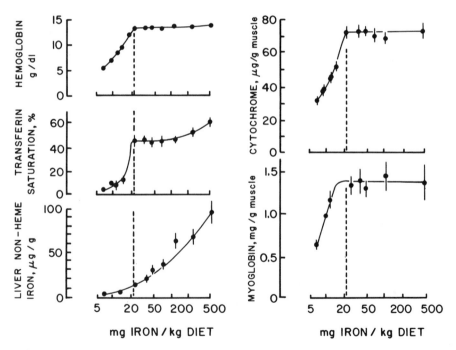

FIG. 9. Effects of various levels of dietary iron deficiency in growing rats on various iron-dependent variables in liver, blood, and muscle (mean ± SEM). (Reproduced from ref. 68 with permission from the *American Journal of Clinical Nutrition*, © 1980.)

the electron influx into the mitochondria but also to the regeneration of cyto-plasmic NAD^+, essential for glycolysis (30,57,71,72). As a result of these limitations in functional mitochondrial oxidative capacity and glycolytic activity, alternative cytoplasmic NAD^+ regeneration, which is indispens-able for extramitochondrial ATP production, must occur in muscle. One way to achieve such regeneration is through the increased utilization of glu-cose and pyruvate via lactate, resulting in increased glucose utilization, lac-tate turnover with greater recycling through glucose, and lactic acidosis. These phenomena have been implicated in the limitations exhibited by iron-deficient rats even when performing submaximal exercise (40,71–74). Endocrine responses to exercise (elevations in glucagon, cortisol, epineph-rine, and norepinephrine) in favor of neoglucogenesis and glucogenolysis have been demonstrated in the anemic dog when compared to the nonanemic state (75). In humans, Gardner et al. (50) demonstrated a progressive lactic acidosis in direct proportion to the severity of the anemia and inversely pro-portional to maximal aerobic capacity in human volunteers performing max-imal exercise tests.

Recently, a series of studies that measured the impact of iron deficiency on maximal or near-maximal effort and endurance capacity demonstrated the relative importance of muscle dysfunction in iron deficiency. The prac-tical importance of these studies relates to the fact that most human physical work is submaximal (at around 40% of VO_2max) and demands various degrees of endurance.

These studies gave rise to the α-glycerophosphate hypothesis as the cause of impaired muscle function and lactic acidosis in iron deficiency. The independence of muscle dysfunction from anemia in iron deficiency was clearly demonstrated by Finch et al. (57), who reported that iron-deficient rats performed poorly on standardized strenuous exercise tests even when they were transfused to the same hemoglobin levels as iron-sufficient animals. They also demonstrated that when iron therapy was pro-vided, work performance improved within 4 days, concomitant with a rise in the activity of the α-glycerophosphate oxidative system. Subsequent studies exploring endurance capacity in iron-deficient rats (30,55,56) pro-vided evidence that muscle bioenergetic dysfunction in this animal is pri-marily responsible for alterations in exercise endurance, while the reduc-tion in maximal aerobic power (VO_2max) is primarily the consequence of impaired oxygen delivery to muscle, resulting from reduced hemoglobin concentration. It would appear that reductions in endurance appear early in progressive iron deficiency and are more severe (76) than limitations in maximal aerobic power. The response pattern to iron repletion suggests that endurance recovers more slowly than VO_2max (30) (Fig. 10). Physical training appears to stimulate the activities of non-iron-dependent enzymes in the tricarboxylic acid cycle of iron-deficient rats, while it has no effect in iron-sufficient animals (77,78). This adaptation increases muscle oxidative capacity, improves lactate homeostasis, and enhances the response to energy demands for endurance in the face of adequate oxygen delivery systems.

Impaired muscle function appears to be subject to iron deficiency at four different key points (Fig. 11). While all four probably are in play simultaneously, each contributes to a different degree depending upon exercise demands. Changes in general metabolic fuel utilization, favoring glucose dependence, appear to be induced by iron deficiency, with loss of metabolic efficiency as a consequence.

Few of the metabolic alterations demonstrated in the iron-deficient rat have been corroborated in the human. Although strong evidence exists for excessive lactic acidemia, as well as some indications of a beneficial effect of iron therapy beyond correction of hemoglobin, evidence for decreased endurance and rapid response to iron therapy is lacking (79,80). Moreover, studies on human skeletal muscle from severely chronic iron-deficient individuals have failed to demonstrate changes similar to those well documented in rats (81).

The role of "anemia" and of iron deficiency in the more general metabolic effects demonstrated in animals needs to be defined in humans, including the sympathetic–norepinephrine and thyroid dysfunction upon which many of the iron–energy and thermoregulation interactions are based (37,82).

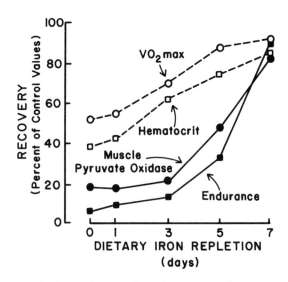

FIG. 10. Recovery of VO₂max, hematocrit, endurance capacity, and muscle homogenate pyruvate–malate oxidase activity of iron-deficient rats during dietary iron repletion (mean percentage of each day's control rats). (Reproduced from ref. 30 with permission from the American Physiological Society, © 1982.)

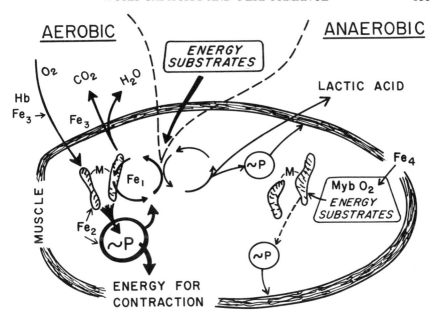

FIG. 11. Schematic representation of sites where iron deficiency induces reduction in muscle function and impairs physical work capacity. Fe_1 = phosphoglycerate shuttle; Fe_2 = oxidative phosphorylation system (muscle oxidative capacity), cytochromes, oxidases, dehydrogenases, Fe–S clusters; Fe_3 = hemoglobin O_2–CO_2 transport; Fe_4 = myoglobin O_2 content.

EFFECTS OF IRON DEFICIENCY AND ITS CORRECTION ON WORK PERFORMANCE AND PRODUCTIVITY

Given the complexity of factors that modulate work performance, most ordinary workday environments do not lend themselves to exploration of the effect of iron deficiency on work capacity and productivity. Two major studies, one in Sri Lanka (41) and the other in Indonesia (38,49,83), have demonstrated the effects of iron deficiency and its correction in work performance and productivity. Both studies included placebo controls and were as free from bias as possible. In Sri Lanka, tea pickers increased their average daily tea weight harvest by 0.3 kg in response to iron administration. The response was greater among those whose hemoglobin concentration was initially < 9 g/dl (1.9 kg/day). This effect occurred "despite the constancy of the physical and psychological environment" provided by rather rigid social concepts of work and labor conditions (41) (Fig. 12). In Indonesia, both rubber tappers (paid by the piece) and weeders (paid by the day) exhibited better work performance and productivity when their hemoglobin levels were higher than their counterparts both throughout the study and as their hematological condition and iron status improved. In the higher hemoglobin group, the measured total latex harvested was almost 16% higher and the

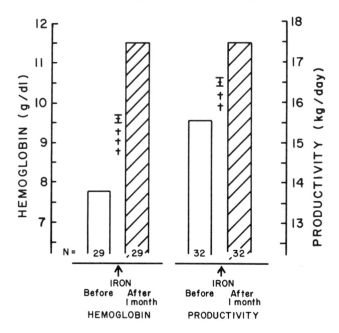

FIG. 12. Effect of oral iron treatment of anemic female tea pickers (Hgb < 9 g/dl) on hemoglobin and kg of tea plucked/day. Bars = mean ± SEM of differences in 1 month time. $p <$ 0.001; $p <$ 0.01. From ref. 41.

area weeded was nearly 15% larger than the totals of their "anemic" counterparts. When the area weeded was expressed on a time basis, the workers with higher hemoglobin values performed better than those with lower hemoglobin values during the first 2 hr of work, although there was no difference in the next 3 hr of the measured work day.

In terms of cost efficiency, the results of both studies justified the economic investment needed to correct iron deficiency. For the rubber tappers, the benefit/cost ratio could be as high as 260:1. In addition, the workers without anemia remained healthier and had less absenteeism than their iron-deficient counterparts (49).

CONCLUSIONS

The maintenance of adequate iron nutrition throughout life seems to favor the achievement of an optimal physical work capacity. In addition, the treatment of iron deficiency produces significant improvements in work capacity and performance. Techniques to achieve both goals are at hand and appear to be highly cost-effective. In the human, the biochemical mechanisms operating at the cellular level in muscle still need clarification. Moreover, the effects of iron deficiency on whole body energy substrate regulation and utilization at rest and during exercise also need to be explored in depth.

REFERENCES

1. Elwood, P. C., Waters, W. E., Greene, W. J. W., and Sweetnam, P. (1969): Symptoms and circulating hemoglobin level. *J. Chron. Dis.*, 21:615–628.
2. United Nations (1987): First Report on the World Nutrition Situation. United Nations Administrative Committee on Coordination—Subcommittee on Nutrition, Rome, November 1987.
3. Viteri, F. E., Alvarado, J., Luthringer, D., and Wood, R. P. II (1968): Hematological changes in protein calorie malnutrition. *Vitamins Hormones,* 27:573–614.
4. Viteri, F. E. (1981): Primary protein–energy malnutrition. Biochemical and metabolic changes. In: *Textbook of Pediatric Nutrition,* edited by R. M. Suskind. Raven Press, New York, pp. 189–215.
5. Parsons, C. G., and Wright, F. H. (1939): Circulatory function in the anemias of children. I. Effect of anemia on exercise tolerance and vital capacity. *Am. J. Dis. Child.,* 57:15–28.
6. Vellar, O. D., and Hermansen, L. (1971): Physical performance and hematological parameters. *Acta Med. Scand.,* suppl 522.
7. Davies, C. T. M. (1973): Physiological responses to exercise in East African children. II. The effects of schistosomiasis, anaemia and malnutrition. *J. Trop. Pediatr.,* 19:115–119.
8. Cullumbine, H. (1949/1950): Hemoglobin concentration and physical fitness. *J. Appl. Physiol.,* 2:274.
9. Gandra, Y. R., and Bradfield, R. B. (1971): Energy expenditure and oxygen handling efficiency of anemic schoolchildren. *Am. J. Clin. Nutr.,* 24:1451–1456.
10. Buzina, R., Grgic, Z., Jusic, M., Sapunar, J., Milanovic, N., and Brubacher, G. (1982): Nutritional status and physical working capacity. *Hum. Nutr. Clin. Nutr.,* 36C:429–438.
11. Powers, H. J., Bates, C. J., Lamb, W. H., Singh, J., Gelman, W., and Webb, E. (1985): Effects of a multivitamin and iron supplement on running performance in Gambian children. *Hum. Nutr. Clin. Nutr.,* 39C:427–437.
12. Davies, C. T. M., Chukweumaka, A. C., and Van Haaren, J. P. M. (1973): Iron deficiency anaemia: its effect on maximum aerobic power and responses to exercise in African males aged 17–40 years. *Clin. Sci.,* 44:555–562.
13. Viteri, F. E., and Torun, B. (1974): Anaemia and physical work capacity. *Clin. Haematol.,* 3:609–626.
14. Ohira, Y., Edgerton, V. R., Gardner, G. W., Senewiratne, B., Barnard, R. J., and Simpson, D. R. (1979): Work capacity, heart rate and blood lactate responses to iron treatment. *Br. J. Haematol.,* 41:365–372.
15. Astrand, P. O., and Rodahl, K. (1986): Physical performance. In: *Textbook of Work Physiology,* 3rd ed., Chap. 7. McGraw-Hill, New York, pp. 295–353.
16. Viteri, F. E. (1971): Considerations on the effect of nutrition on the body composition and physical working capacity of young Guatemalan adults. In: *Amino Acid Fortification of Foods,* edited by N. S. Scrimshaw and A. Altschul. MIT Press, Cambridge, MA, pp. 350–375.
17. Spurr, G. B., Barac-Nieto, M., and Maksud, M. G. (1977): Productivity and maximal oxygen consumption in sugar can cutters. *Am. J. Clin. Nutr.,* 30:316–321.
18. Beutler, E. (1980): Iron. In: Modern Nutrition in Health and Disease, 6th ed., edited by R. S. Goodhart and M. E. Shils. Lea & Febiger, Philadelphia, pp. 324–349.
19. Edgerton, V. R., Bryant, S. L., Gillespie, C. A., and Gardner, G. W. (1972): Iron deficiency anemia and physical performance and activity of rats. *J. Nutr.,* 102:381–400.
20. McCall, M. G., Newman, G. E., O'Brien, J. R. P., Valberg, L. S., and Witts, L. J. (1962): Studies in iron metabolism. I. The experimental production of iron deficiency in the growing rat. *Br. J. Nutr.,* 16:297–304.
21. Pollitt, E., Viteri, F., Saco-Pollit, C., and Leibel, R. L. (1982): Functional aspects of iron deficiency. In: *Iron deficiency: brain biochemistry and behavior,* edited by R. Leibel and E. Pollitt. Raven Press, New York, pp. 195–208.
22. Chandra, R. K., and Saraya, A. K. (1975): Impaired immunocompetence associated with iron deficiency. *J. Pediatr.,* 86:899–902.
23. Keusch, G. T., Wilson, C. S., and Waksal, S. D. (1983): Nutrition, host defenses and the lymphoid

system. In: *Advances in Host Defense Mechanisms*, Vol. 2, edited by A. S. Fauci and J. I. Gallin. Raven Press, New York, pp. 275–359.

24. Walter, T. (1989): Iron and infection. In: *Dietary Iron: Birth to Two Years*, edited by L. J. Filer, Jr. Raven Press, New York.

25. Basta, S. S., Soekirman, Karyadi, D., and Scrimshaw, N. S. (1979): Iron deficiency anemia and the productivity of adult males in Indonesia. *Am. J. Clin. Nutr.*, 32:916–925.

26. Mata, L. J., Urrutia, J. J., Albertazzi, C., Pellecer, O., and Arellano, E. (1972): Influence of recurrent infections on nutrition and growth of children in Guatemala. *Am. J. Clin. Nutr.*, 25:1267–1275.

27. Martorell, R., and Yarbrough, C. (1983): The energy cost of diarrheal diseases and other common illnesses in children. In: *Diarrhea and Nutrition*, edited by L. C. Chen and N. S. Scrimshaw. Plenum Publishing Corp., New York.

28. Bender-Gotze Ch., Ludwig, U., Schafer, K. H., Heinrich, H. C., and Oppitz, K. H. (1976): Cytochemische Knochenmarksbefunde und diagnostiche $^{59}FE^{2+}$—Absorption wahren des akuten und chronischen Infektes im Kindesalter. *Monatsschr. Kinderheilkd., 124:305–316.*

29. Bothwell, T. H., Charlton, R. W., Cook, J. D., and Finch, C. A. (1979): *Iron Metabolism in Man* Blackwell Scientific, Oxford, pp. 1–576.

30. Davies, K. J. A., Maguire, J. J., Brooks, G. A., Dallman, P. R., and Packer, L. (1982): Muscle mitochondrial bioenergetics, oxygen supply and work capacity during dietary iron deficiency and repletion. *Am. J. Physiol.*, 242:E418–E427.

31. Martinez-Torres, C., Cubeddu, L., Dillman, E., et al. (1984): Effect of exposure to low temperature on normal and iron-deficient subjects. *Am. J. Physiol.*, 246:R380–R383.

32. Walter, T. (1989): Effect of iron deficiency anemia on infant psychomotor development. In: *Dietary Iron: Birth to Two Years*, edited by L. J. Filer, Jr. Raven Press, New York.

33. Voorhees, M. L., Stuart, M. J., Stockman, J. A., and Oski, F. A. (1975): Iron deficiency anemia and increased urinary norepinephrine excretion. *J. Pediatr.*, 86:542–547.

34. Beard, J., and Borel, M. (1988): Iron deficiency and thermoregulation. *Nutr. Today*, Sept/Oct:41–45.

35. Dillman, E., Johnson, D. G., Martin, J., Mackler, B., and Finch, C. (1979): Catecholamine elevation in iron deficiency. *Am. J. Physiol.*, 237:R297–R300.

36. Dillman, E., Gale, C. H., Green, W., Johnson, D. G., Mackler, B., and Finch, C. A. (1980): Hypothermia in iron deficiency due to altered triiodothyronine metabolism. *Am. J. Physiol.*, 239:R377–R381.

37. Beard, J., Tobin, B., and Smith, S. M. (1988): Norepinephrine turnover in iron deficiency at three environmental temperatures. *Am. J. Physiol.*, 255:R90–R96.

38. Edgerton, V. R., Ohira, Y., Gardner, G. W., Senewiratne, B. Effects of iron deficiency anemia on voluntary activities in rats and humans. (1982): In: *Iron Deficiency: Brain Biochemistry and Behavior*, edited by E. Pollitt and R. L. Leibel. Raven Press, New York, pp. 141–160.

39. Mackler, B., Person, R., Miller, L. R., and Finch, C. A. (1979): Iron deficiency in the rat: effects on phenylalanine metabolism. *Pediatr. Res.*, 13:1010–1011.

40. Edgerton, V. R., Diamond, L. B., and Olson, J. (1977): Voluntary activity, cardiovascular and muscular responses to anemia in rats. *J. Nutr.*, 107:1595–1601.

41. Edgerton, V. R., Gardner, G. W., Ohira, Y., Gunawardena, K. A., and Senewiratne, B. (1979): Iron deficiency anemia and its effect on worker productivity and activity patterns. *Br. Med. J.*, 2:1546–1549.

42. Viteri, F. E., and Torun, B. (1981): Nutrition, physical activity and growth. In: *The Biology of Normal Human Growth*, edited by M. Ritzen. Raven Press, New York, pp. 265–273.

43. Bowering, J., and Norton, G. F. (1981): Relationship between iron status and exercise in male and female growing rats. *J. Nutr.*, 111:1648–1657.

44. Strause, L., Hegenauer, J., and Saltman, P. (1983): Effects of exercise on iron metabolism in rats. *Nutr. Res.*, 3:79–89.

45. Perkkio, M. V., Jansson, L. T., Henderson, S., Refino, C., Brooks, G. A., and Dallman, P. R. (1985): Work performance in the iron-deficient rat: improved endurance with exercise training. *Am. J. Physiol.*, 249:E306–E311.

46. Willis, W. T., Brooks, G. A., Henderson, S. A., and Dallman, P. R. (1987): Effects of iron deficiency and training on mitochondrial enzymes in skeletal muscle. *J. Appl. Physiol.*, 62:2442–2446.

47. Willis, W. T., Dallman, P. R., and Brooks, G. A. (1988): Physiological and biochemical correlates of increased work in trained iron-deficient rats. *J. Appl. Physiol.*, 65:256–263.

48. Viteri, F. E. (1976): Definition of the nutrition problem in the labor force. In: *Nutrition and Agricultural Development—Significance and Potential for the Tropics,* edited by N. S. Scrimshaw and M. Behar. Plenum Press, New York, pp. 87–98.
49. Basta, S. (1974): Iron deficiency anemia in adult males and work capacity. Sc.D. Thesis, Massachusetts Institute of Technology.
50. Gardner, G. W., Edgerton, V. R., Senewiratne, B., Barnard, R. J., and Ohira, Y. (1977): Physical work capacity and metabolic stress in subjects with iron deficiency anemia. *Am. J. Clin. Nutr.,* 30:910–917.
51. Celsing, F., Svedenhag, J., Pihlstedt, P., and Ekblom, E. (1987): Effects of anemia and stepwise-induced polycythaemia on maximal aerobic power in individuals with high and low hemoglobin concentrations. *Acta Physiol. Scand.,* 129:47–54.
52. Celsing, F., and Ekblom, B. (1986): Anemia causes a relative decrease in blood lactate concentration during exercise. *Eur. J. Appl., Physiol.,* 55:74–78.
53. Wrane, B., and Woodson, R. D. (1973): A graded treadmill test for rats: maximal work performance in normal and anemic animals. *J. Appl. Physiol.,* 34:732–735.
54. Ohira, Y., Koziol, B. J., Edgerton, V. R., and Brooks, G. A. (1981): Oxygen consumption and work capacity in iron-deficient anemia rats. *J. Nutr.,* 111:17–25.
55. Davies, K. J. A., Donovan, C. M., Refino, C. J., Brooks, G. A., Packer, L., and Dallman, P. R. (1984): Distinguishing effects of anemia and muscle iron deficiency on exercise bioenergetics in the rat. *Am. J. Physiol.,* 246:E535–E543.
56. Perkkio, M. V., Jansson, L. T., Brooks, G. A., Refino, C. J., and Dallman, P. R. (1985): Work performance in iron deficiency of increasing severity. *J. Appl. Physiol.,* 58:1477–1480.
57. Finch, C. A., Miller, L. R., Inamdar, A. R., Person, R., Seiler, K., and Mackler, B. (1976): Physiological and biochemical studies of muscle dysfunction. *J. Clin. Invest.,* 58:447–453.
58. Astrand, P. O., and Rodahl, K. (1986): Body fluids, blood and circulation, and respiration. In: *Textbook of Work Physiology,* 3rd ed., Chaps. 4 and 5. McGraw-Hill, New York, pp. 127–272.
59. Ekblom, B., Huot, R., Stein, E. M., and Thorstensson, A. (1975): Effect of changes in arterial oxygen content on circulation and physical performance. *J. Appl. Physiol.,* 39:71–77.
60. Torrance, J., Jacobs, P., Restrepo, A., Eschbach, J., Lenfant, C., and Finch, C. A. (1970): Intraerythrocytic adaptation to anemia. *N. Engl. J. Med.,* 382:165–169.
61. Woodson, R. D., Wills, R. E., and Lenfant, C. (1978): Effect of acute and established anemia on O_2 transport at rest, submaximal and maximal work. *J. Appl. Physiol.,* 44:36–43.
62. Celsing, F., Nystrom, J., Pihlstedt, P., Werner, B., and Ekblom, B. (1986): Effect of long-term anemia and retransfusion on cnetal circulation during exercise. *J. Appl. Physiol.,* 61:1358–1362.
63. Beutler, E. (1957): Iron enzymes in iron deficiency. I. Cytochrome c. *Am. J. Med. Sci.,* 234:517–519.
64. Dallman, P. R., and Schwartz, H. C. (1965): Distribution of cytochrome c and myoglobin in rats with dietary iron deficiency. *Pediatrics,* 35:677–686.
65. Dallman, P. R., and Schwartz, H. C. (1965): Myoglobin and cytochrome responses during repair of iron deficiency in the rat. *J. Clin. Invest.,* 44:1631–1638.
66. Dallman, P. R. (1974): Tissue effects of iron deficiency. In: *Iron in Biochemistry and Medicine,* edited by M. Worwood and A. Jacobs. Academic Press, New York, pp. 437–475.
67. World Health Organization (1972): Nutritional anemias. WHO Technical Report Series 503.
68. Siimes, M. A., Refino, C., and Dallman, P. R. (1980): Manifestation of iron deficiency of various levels of dietary iron intake. *Am. J. Clin. Nutr.,* 33:570–574.
69. Koziol, B. J., Ohira, Y., Simpson, D. R., and Edgerton, V. R. (1978): Biochemical skeletal muscle and hematological profiles of moderate and severely iron deficient and anemic adult rats. *J. Nutr.,* 108:1306–1314.
70. Maguire, J. J., Davies, K. J. A., Dallman, P. R., and Packer, L. (1982): Effects of dietary iron deficiency on iron–sulfur proteins and bioenergetic functions of skeletal muscle mitochondria. *Biomed. Biophys. Acta.,* 679:210–220.
71. Finch, C. A., Gollnick, P. D., Hlastala, M. P., Miller, L. R., Dillman, E., and Mackler, B. (1979): Lactic acidosis as a result of iron deficiency. *J. Clin. Invest.,* 64:129–137.
72. McLane, J. A., Fell, R. D., McKay, R. H., Winder, W. W., Brown, E. B., and Holloszy, J. O. (1981): Physiological and biochemical effects of iron deficiency on rat skeletal muscle. *Am. J. Physiol.,* 241:C47–C54.
73. Henderson, S. A., Dallman, P. R., and Brooks, G. A. (1986): Glucose turnover and oxidation are increased in the iron-deficient anemic rat. *Am. J. Physiol.,* 250:E414–E421.

74. Brooks, G. A., Henderson, S. A., and Dallman, P. R. (1987): Increased glucose dependence in resting, iron deficient rats. *Am. J. Physiol.,* 253:E461–E466.
75. Wasserman, D. H., Lavina, H., Lickley, A., and Vranic, M. (1985): Effect of hematocrit reduction on hormonal and metabolic responses to exercise. *J. Appl. Physiol.,* 58:1257–1262.
76. Davies, K. J. A., Packer, L., and Brooks, G. A. (1981): Biochemical adaptation of mitochondria, muscle and whole animal respiration to endurance training: mitochondrial respiration and exercise energetics. *Arch. Biochem. Biophys.,* 209:539–554.
77. Willis, W. T., Brooks, G. A., Henderson, S. A., and Dallman, P. R. (1987): Effects of iron deficiency and training on mitochondrial enzymes in skeletal muscle. *J. Appl. Physiol.,* 62:2442–2446.
78. Willis, W. T., Dallman, P. R., and Brooks, G. A. (1988): Physiological and biochemical correlates of increased work in trained iron-deficient rats. *J. Appl. Physiol.,* 65:256–263.
79. Ohira, Y., Edgerton, V. R., Gardner, G. W., Senewiratne, B., and Simpson, D. R. (1978): Non-hemoglobin related effects on heart rate in iron deficiency anemia. *Nutr. Rep. Int.,* 18:647–651.
80. Charlton, R. W., Derman, D., Skikne, B., et al. (1977): Anemia, iron deficiency and exercise: extended studies in human subjects. *Clin. Sci. Mol. Med.,* 53:537–541.
81. Celsing, F., Ekblom, B., Sylven, C., Everett, J., and Astrad, P. O. (1988): Effects of chronic iron deficiency anemia on myoglobin content, enzyme activity, and capillary density in human skeletal muscle. *Acta Med. Scand.,* 223:451–457.
82. Beard, J., Green, W., Miller, L., and Finch, C. A. (1984): Effect of iron-deficiency anemia on hormone levels and thermoregulation during cold exposure. *Am. J. Physiol.,* 247:R114–R119.
83. Scrimshaw, N. S. (1984): Functional consequences of iron deficiency in human populations. *J. Nutr. Sci. Vitaminol.,* 30:47–63.

Dietary Iron: Birth to Two Years,
edited by L. J. Filer, Jr.
Raven Press, Ltd., New York © 1989.

Effect of Iron Deficiency Anemia on Infant Psychomotor Development

Tomas Walter

Institute of Nutrition and Food Technology, University of Chile, 15138 Santiago 11, Chile

Heralded by the pioneering work of Oski and Honig a decade ago (1), more than a dozen studies have addressed the effects of iron deficiency on cognitive development during infancy. The inherent difficulties of identifying intervening variables in the complex field of mental development, coupled in some cases with poor experimental design, have mitigated against making significant headway.

Two recent studies, one performed in Costa Rica by Lozoff et al. (2) and the other in Santiago de Chile by our group (3), have controlled for many of the uncertainties that have precluded drawing firm conclusions from previous work. The two studies, both initiated in 1982–1983, produced similar results, thereby providing considerable strength to the conclusions. The similarities in findings are remarkable in spite of the fact that there were important differences in study design and that the research was carried out by two independent investigators in two distant regions.

The effects of iron deficiency on infant behavior were evaluated in Chile in a study completed in 1985 that was performed in conjunction with a field trial of fortified infant foods (3).

MATERIALS AND METHODS

Briefly, a cohort of healthy, full-term infants from a community clinic in the city of Santiago were enrolled at 3 months of age in a food fortification study and followed to 12 months of age with monthly clinic checkups and weekly home visits by a nurse. Complete anthropometric, nutritional, morbidity, and socioeconomic data were collected. Infants who had been weaned from the breast by 3 months received either iron-fortified cow's milk or non-iron-fortified milk provided at no cost by the clinic. Infants who continued to be breast-fed at 3 months of age were assigned to one of two groups. The first group received a heme iron-fortified cereal in addition to normal nonmilk foods, and the second group received the same diet without iron fortification.

Because the assignment to iron fortification was random, all confounding factors other than iron status were essentially offset by this design.

Approximately 100 infants were entered in each of the four groups, with each group having an attrition rate of about 20% over the 9 months of follow-up due mainly to migration. At 9 and 12 months of age, venipunctures for a full hematological assessment were performed. Parents were invited to enroll their infants at 12 months of age in the psychological study. After informed consent was obtained, psychological testing was initiated 7 to 10 days following the 12-month checkup.

Assessment of iron status at 12 months of age permitted a preliminary classification of subjects based on hemoglobin, mean corpuscular volume, and free erythrocyte protoporphyrin. The first Bayley Scales of Infant Development (BSID) were performed at this time. Within each initial iron status group, infants were randomly assigned to receive iron sulfate drops or placebo for 10 days, when the BSID was repeated. At this time, all infants received iron sulfate drops to provide at 3 to 5 mg/kg body weight/day in two divided doses for 75 days, at the end of which the BSID was readministered and iron status assessments repeated.

All of the Bayley tests were administered by the same psychologist, who was unaware of the iron status of the infants, and the therapy assignment, facts also unknown to the mother.

The BSID is an accepted tool to evaluate psychomotor development from age 3 to 30 months (4). The Bayley Scales consist of (a) a mental scale evaluating functions related to the basic foundation for cognition such as language acquisition and abstract thinking; (b) a motor or psychomotor scale relating to gross motor abilities such as coordination, body balance, and walking. Both scales are age-adjusted to give an index of mental and psychomotor development (MDI and PDI, respectively) very much like an IQ with a mean of 100 and a standard deviation of 16; (c) the Infant Behavior Record (IBR), based on clinical observation by the psychologist, does not yield a score. Although the test has drawbacks, such as its global nature and poor IQ predictability (5), it is well known, reproducible, reliable, and generally accepted as a good measure of behavior in infancy.

The aims of our study were to provide answers to the following questions: (a) What is the severity of iron deficiency necessary to affect behavior? (b) What is the effect of the duration of iron deficiency? (c) Is short-term iron therapy (before correction of anemia) effective? (d) How reversible are the behavioral changes after long-term iron therapy (enough to correct anemia)? (e) What are the specific areas of mental or motor processes most affected? (f) What are the possible associations of developmental deficits with behavior patterns?

Criteria for classification of the infants into three groups—anemic, control, and nonanemic iron-deficient (NAID)—are shown in Table 1. The broad heterogeneity of the NAID group prompted its reclassification into three grades of severity: Grade 1 (iron depleted), all measures normal except for serum ferritin (< 10 µg/L); Grade 2 (nonresponder), one to four abnormal values but with a therapeutic response (hemoglobin: < 1.0 g/dl); and Grade 3 (responder), zero to four abnormal values and/or a therapeutic response (hemoglobin: > 1.0 g/dl).

RESULTS AND DISCUSSION

Hematological Data

Complete hematological evaluation was performed in 189 infants at 9 months of age (when no BSIDs were done), and in 196 infants at 12 and 15 months. The final classification of the infants and mean values for hematological measures are shown in Table 2. Our controls complied with the most stringent criteria to define iron repletion, and the subclassification of NAID succeeded in segregating degrees of severity noted in the progression of iron status measurements (Table 3).

TABLE 1. *Classification criteria for iron nutritional status*

Control	Hemoglobin ≥ 11.0 g/dl
	Mean corpuscular volume: ≥ 70 fl
	Serum iron/total iron binding capacity: $\geq 10\%$
	Free erythrocyte protoporphyrin: < 100 µg of zinc protoporphyrin/dl
	Serum ferritin: ≥ 10 µg/L
	Response to iron therapy: Hgb < 1.0 g/dl
Anemic	Hemoglobin: < 11.0 g/dl and two or more abnormal biochemical measures
NAID[a]	Hemoglobin: ≥ 11 g/dl
	One or more abnormal biochemical measures or a response to iron therapy: hemoglobin ≥ 1.0 g/dl

[a]NAID: nonanemic iron-deficient infants.

TABLE 2. *Iron nutritional status at 12 months (mean $\pm$ SD)*

	Control (N = 30)	Anemic (N = 39)	NAID[a] (N = 127)
Hemoglobin (g/dl)	12.7 ± 0.8	10.0 ± 0.9	12.1 ± 0.7
Fe/TIBC (%)[b]	16.7 ± 6.3	6.8 ± 2.9	12.2 ± 0.7
FEP[c]	78 ± 13	195 ± 103	108 ± 33
Serum ferritin[d] (µg/L)	19.8 (12–34)	5.4 (3–9.8)	11.9 (6–24)

[a]NAID = nonanemic iron-deficient.
[b]Fe/TIBC = serum iron/total iron binding capacity.
[c]FEP = free erythrocyte protoporphyrin (µg of ZPP/dl of red blood cells).
[d]Geometric mean and range: 1 SD.

Development Scores

A total of 576 BSIDs were administered. Mean MDI was 102.4 $\pm$ 9, and mean PDI was 98.1 $\pm$ 11. Although there was a significant difference between MDI and PDI in the study population as a whole, both distributions were symmetric (Fig. 1). This population was biased by design since we had selected healthy infants from a closely followed cohort. We purposely excluded confounding influences in the population and environment by longitudinally following a cohort of infants in an optimal state of health, with

TABLE 3. *Subclassification of nonanemic iron-deficient infants*

	Grade 1 (iron-depleted)	Grade 2 (nonresponder)	Grade 3 (responder)
Hemoglobin (g/dl)	12.9 $\pm$ 0.6	12.3 $\pm$ 0.7	11.7 $\pm$ 0.5
Fe/TIBC (%)[a]	14.8 $\pm$ 3.6	12.3 $\pm$ 0.7	11.7 $\pm$ 0.5
FEP[b]	81 $\pm$ 12	107 $\pm$ 30	115 $\pm$ 38
Serum ferritin[c] (μg/L)	7.5 (6.7–8.2)	15 (7.7–27)	9 (4.1–20)

[a]Fe/TIBC = serum iron/total iron binding capacity.
[b]FEP = free erythrocyte protoporphyrin (μg of ZPP/dl of red blood cells).
[c]Geometric mean and range: 1 SD.

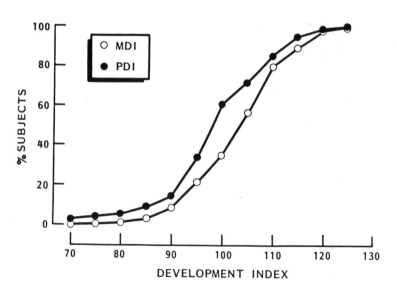

FIG. 1. Cumulative plot of all measures of developmental indices. Note the leftward shift of PDI with conservation of symmetry at all index levels.

the exception of iron nutritional status. Furthermore, the infant's iron status was determined randomly by random assignment to iron-fortified foods. The proximity of the scores to the U.S. norm and the symmetry of the BSID distribution is likely a consequence of this design, which eliminated confounding low performances usually present in disadvantaged populations.

Effect of Iron Status on Developmental Scores

It is clear that a decrease in hemoglobin leading to anemia is required in order to affect mental and psychomotor development scores (Fig. 2). The performance of the NAID infants as a whole was indistinguishable from that of control infants. None of the NAID subclassifications was successful in showing differences (Fig. 3). Even infants in group three, i.e., infants who were nonanemic and responded to the therapeutic trial (and who could there-

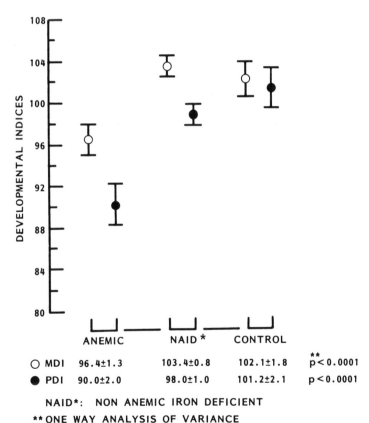

FIG. 2.   Effect of anemia age 12 months on developmental indices. Anemics show a significant fall in PDI and MDI, whereas NAID and controls are not significantly different.

fore technically be defined as anemic), did not show any tendency toward lower scores.

Although a difference between MDI and PDI was present in all groups, this difference seemed to be of smaller magnitude in the control group, where mental and motor performance appeared to be better balanced (Fig. 3). As iron deficiency progressed, motor performance was more affected than mental index, as seen by the divergence of the mean values. Explanations for this phenomenon remain conjectural.

If the effect of iron deficiency on behavior was mediated by metabolic processes dependent on the presence of iron, overt anemia might be necessary to disclose these effects. Siimes et al. (8) showed in an animal model fed graded amounts of iron that tissue heme proteins were not affected until saturation of transferrin fell significantly. Hemoglobin, tissue cytochrome C, and myoglobin concentration decreased steadily thereafter, demonstrating that availability of iron to the erythroid marrow is limited concomitantly to other tissues. Changes in iron stores (liver non-heme iron) did not influence hemoglobin level or tissue heme iron proteins. In humans, the stage known as "iron deficient erythropoiesis," when iron availability becomes a

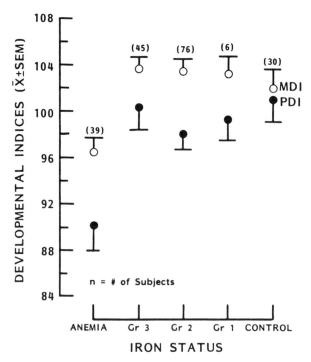

FIG. 3. MDI–PDI according to iron status at age 12 months. Different grades of NAID failed to show any tendency toward lower scores, even in NAID Grade 3, which could technically be classified as "anemic." (n) = number of subjects.

limiting factor for hemoglobin synthesis, corresponds to the moment when hemoglobin concentration begins to decrease, presumably along with other tissue iron proteins.

However, the stage of overt anemia is reached later, when hemoglobin values fall below 11.0 g/dl in the infant. Anemia ensues, therefore, after a rather protracted and severe period of iron deficiency, ensuring significant depletion of tissue iron proteins. Milder iron deficit may fall short of achieving sufficient tissue depletion so as not to be reflected in behavior. On the other hand, the psychological tests available for infants may be too crude to identify subtle deficits. These considerations may help explain the absence of differences in cognitive effects seen in the nonanemic responder population (subclassification NAID Grade 3), which conceivably corresponds to a group of infants with limited hemoglobin synthesis, soon to become anemic.

Effect of Hemoglobin on Development Scores

Examination of MDI and PDI based on hemoglobin concentration as the most common indicator of iron status defined a sigmoid distribution with hemoglobin intervals of 0.5 g/dl (Fig. 4). Here, three groups were identified: those < 10.5 g/dl; those > 11.0 g/dl; and an intermediate group at 10.5–10.9 g/dl. All were statistically distinct from each other by pairwise and ANOVA comparisons. Thus, among anemic infants, hemoglobin concentration is correlated with performance, so that infants with moderate anemia (hemoglobin of 8.4–10.4 g/dl) have significantly lower developmental scores than those with mild degrees of anemia (hemoglobin of 10.5–10.9 g/dl). These, in turn, have poorer developmental scores than infants with hemoglobin concentration > 11.0 g/dl with no graded improvements seen at higher hemoglobin levels.

Effect of Duration of Anemia

For this purpose, we studied the effect of iron status at 9 months of age on developmental indices measured at 12 months. Indices distributed according to hemoglobin concentration at age 9 months, i.e., 3 months before the BSID tests were performed, showed a cutoff value at 10.5 g/dl. To determine further the effect of duration of anemia, infants who were anemic at both 9 and 12 months, and whose anemia had a duration of 3 or more months ($n = 19$), were compared with those who were anemic at 12 but not at 9 months, i.e., those whose anemia was presumed to be present for less than 3 months ($n = 16$). Of the 39 infants who were anemic at 12 months, only 35 had hemoglobin concentrations determined at 9 months. Those infants who were anemic for more than 3 months had significantly lower development indices than those who were anemic less than 3 months ($p <$

0.05). Moreover, those infants nonanemic at 9 months fell mostly in the intermediate hemoglobin range of 10.5–10.9 g/dl at 12 months, where development indices were less severely affected. Thus, infants who were not anemic at 9 months tended to have milder anemia at 12 months. Of the 14 infants in the intermediate hemoglobin group at 12 months, 10 (71%) were not anemic at 9 months. Of the 21 infants who fell below the intermediate hemoglobin level, only 6 (29%) were not anemic at 9 months ($p < 0.015$). It is apparent from these results that as anemia is prolonged, and consequently of greater intensity, developmental indices also become more adversely affected.

In summary, infants whose anemia lasted more than 3 months had significantly lower scores than anemic infants whose hemoglobin levels were in the normal range 3 months earlier. Infants without anemia but with marginal iron status at 9 months of age were those who at 12 months of age fell in the intermediate group (hemoglobin of 10.5–10.9 g/dl), i.e., infants who had anemia of shorter duration and less severity, associated with milder psychomotor derangements. If this intermediate group of infants were to continue with an iron-deficient diet, it is likely that their anemia would increase in duration (and severity) and their psychomotor performance would presumably deteriorate further. Unfortunately, these two characteristics of anemia,

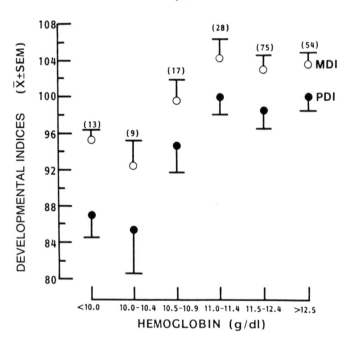

FIG. 4. MDI–PDI according to hemoglobin at age 12 months. An intermediate group (hemoglobin of 10.5–10.9 g/dl) is distinctly different in PDI and MDI from groups with < 10.4 and > 11.0 g/dl of hemoglobin. (n) = number of subjects.

i.e., duration and severity, could not be completely individualized within the current design.

Effect of Iron Therapy

The developmental scores of infants given 10 days of oral ferrous sulfate were compared to those given placebo. Both groups demonstrated similar and significant improvement of developmental indices in mental and psychomotor scales, regardless of prior iron status or therapy. Average improvements were 4.4 to 8.9 points. After 3 months of iron therapy, even though anemia was reversed in all infants and hematological measures of iron status were completely corrected in 11 of the 39 formerly anemic infants, no significant improvement was detected in the developmental scores at 12 and 15 months. Control and NAID infants showed no significant changes in MDI or PDI. Neither paired-t comparisons within groups (highest $p = 0.18$ for controls) nor ANOVA of the differences of scores between groups showed significant changes from baseline BSID scores.

Short-term therapy, before anemia was reversed, was aimed at immediately correcting the availability of iron to processes of neurotransmitter metabolism that are hypothesized to mediate the behavioral derangements seen during iron deficiency (9). In a previous study (10), we found significant improvement in the developmental scores of anemic infants after 10 days of oral iron therapy, whereas no change was noted in nonanemic infants. However, doubts were raised about the interpretation of those results, since the study did not include placebo-treated infants, and neither regression to the mean nor "ceiling" effects could be excluded. In the current double-blind study, the increase in developmental scores among anemic infants treated with iron for 10 days was not significantly greater than that found among placebo-treated anemic infants. The same was true for infants in the other iron status groups. These findings stress the importance of appropriate controls. Similar results were reported recently by Lozoff from Costa Rica (2), supporting the assertion that short-term iron therapy does not exert a change in performance beyond what could be explained by a "practice effect."

After 3 months of iron treatment, most of the infants enrolled in this study had completely corrected their hematological status, and all had reversed their anemia. This stage represents tissue replenishment of iron and ensures renewal of those iron enzymes with turnover times similar to or shorter than hemoglobin. If these tissue iron proteins were responsible for developmental test performance scores, anemic infants would have approached those of their iron-replete peers. Since this did not occur, it is probable that (a) other reactions not directly dependent on iron availability were responsible for the derangements seen; (b) those iron-sensitive behavioral processes may require a longer time for their correction; or (c) they were, in fact, irreversibly damaged.

Specific Patterns of Failure

We have examined the specific test items involved in the raw score that, when normalized for age, yield the developmental index. The MDI scores were encompassed representatively by items 99 to 117 (Table 4) and the corresponding PDI items were 40 to 52 (Table 5). On the mental scale, the items that required comprehension of language but did not involve a visual demonstration were passed significantly by fewer anemic infants than by controls. On the BSID, language development at 12 months was best marked by item 106, "vocalization of bisyllabic words," with differences between anemic infants and controls ($p < 0.01$). The language item 113, "says two words (meaningfully)," was passed by too few infants at 12 months; however, at 15 months, it became significant ($p = 0.005$). At 15 months, item 117, "shows shoes or other clothing or own toy," also became suggestive ($p < 0.07$).

In the psychomotor milestones (Table 5), it appeared that those items relating to balance in the standing position and body control (sits from standing, stands alone, and walks alone) were accomplished by significantly fewer anemic infants than by controls. Differences for items 47 ("stands up from sitting") and 52 ("stands on left foot with help") were not identified at 12 months but became significant at 15 months ($p < 0.05$).

TABLE 4. *Mental scale items at 12 and 15 months: percentage of infants passing*

Description (item no.)	Infants passing (%)		p value[a]
	Anemic	Control	
Pushes car along (99)	56	77	NS[b]
Jabbers expressively (101)	92	93	NS
Uncovers blue box (102)	31	47	NS
Turns book pages (103)	69	83	NS
Pats whistle-doll (in imitation) (104)	44	63	NS
Imitates words (mama, dada) (106)			
At 12 months	13	47	0.01
At 15 months	75	100	0.07
Says two words with meaning (113)			
At 12 months	0	7	NS
At 15 months	42	93	0.005
Shows own shoes, toy, clothing (117)			
At 12 months	0	18	NS
At 15 months	25	60	0.07

[a]Analyzed by χ^2 of absolute numbers.
[b]NS = not significant.

Effect of Iron Status on the Infant Behavior Record (IBR)

Of the 24 items evaluated by the IBR at 12 months, 9 were rated significantly better in control infants than in anemic infants, as shown for responsiveness to the examiner ($p < 0.03$), responsiveness to the mother ($p < 0.0005$), general emotional tone ($p < 0.04$), goal directedness ($p < 0.0005$), attention span ($p < 0.001$), activity ($p < 0.001$), responsiveness to persons ($p < 0.001$), vocalizations ($p < 0.05$), and body motion ($p < 0.002$).

Further analysis of the IBR was performed to associate behavior items related to "test affect" and "task orientation," as suggested by Matheny (11). The test affect combination rated significantly better in the control group than in the anemic group ($p < 0.04$). Those anemic infants with abnormal test affect (14/39) commonly had more scores under the mean for MDI ($p < 0.04$) and PDI ($p < 0.04$), whereas controls showed no differences, probably because very few (3/30) presented an abnormal affect behavior pattern. Abnormal task orientation in the anemic infants (12/39) was markedly associated with MDIs under the mean ($p < 0.01$); however, only a marginal tendency was seen for lower PDIs ($p = 0.09$). Controls showed nonsignificant associations of scores with task orientation, because only 4 of 30 ranked inappropriate task orientation.

These IBR findings expand our previous experience (10) and that of other investigators (6). No appreciable changes were seen in the IBR after therapy, correlating with the lack of change in development index scores. This fact lends support to the hypothesis that the unfavorable behavior pattern of these infants may be a mediator of the poorer BSID performance. If this contention were true, it would probably have affected individual items in a ran-

TABLE 5. *Motor scale items at 12 and 15 months: percentage of infants passing*

Description (item no.)	Infants passing (%)		p value[a]
	Anemic	Control	
Walks with help (42)	85	97	NS[b]
Sits from standing (43)	67	97	0.01
Pat-a-cake (44)	82	97	NS
Stands alone (45)	64	93	0.02
Walks alone (46)	38	67	0.05
Stands up from sitting (47)			
At 12 months	3	7	NS
At 15 months	42	80	0.05
Stands on left foot with help (52)			
At 12 months	0	10	NS
At 15 months	8	40	0.05

[a]Analyzed by χ^2 of absolute numbers.
[b]NS = not significant.

dom fashion. However, in this study, item performance failures have a consistent pattern with preferences for language in the mental items and body balance–coordination in motor skills. The reason for this selective effect remains obscure. Moreover, these findings coincide quite closely with the results of Lozoff (2), who showed similar selective failure patterns using a different study design. While this agreement confirms our findings, it is also worrisome because these findings fail to show consistent improvement after short- or long-term iron therapy.

Comparison Between the Present Study and the Lozoff Study

The study by Lozoff (2) in Costa Rica was also community-based; however, the infants were selected on a door-to-door basis, and a finger prick hematocrit was used to define iron nutritional status. By contrast, the infants in Chile were followed longitudinally during the first year of life, and their iron nutritional status was determined by random assignment to an iron-fortified or non-iron-fortified food. In the Chilean study, the iron fortification assignment was randomized; however, the initial assignment to breast-fed versus early weaning was not random. For breast-fed infants, human milk was the sole source of milk for an average of 275 ± 78 days compared with early weaned infants, for whom the figure was 74 ± 61 days. Nevertheless, human milk was continued with the addition of cow's milk supplements (and other solid foods) in both the breast-fed infants and the early weaned infants for an average of 334 ± 55 and 171 ± 120 days, respectively. However, when iron status was sorted out, the differences in BSID scores between anemic and nonanemic infants persisted.

Like our study, Lozoff's study was double-blind, randomized, and controlled (2). Infants enrolled in the Lozoff study were 12 to 23 months of age ($N = 191$), whereas all infants enrolled in the Chilean study were 12 months of age. This difference was a handicap in one way, because developmental milestones were age-dependent, but an advantage, on the other hand, because some of the motor performances could be examined in the wider span of activities that occur between age 12 and 24 months.

Lozoff's classification of iron status included two overlapping criteria (Table 6). The criterion of hemoglobin level, using a slightly higher value to define nonanemic infants, was predicated on the fact that Hatillo, the community studied, is 1,100 m above sea level.

The level of hemoglobin that defined anemia was lower than the level used in Chile. Iron depletion, iron deficiency, and iron sufficiency were classified using the biochemical indices of percent iron saturation, serum ferritin, and free erythrocyte proporphyrin. Fortunately, classifications of iron status from both community studies could be compared, even though we separated anemia sharply at 11 g/dl of hemoglobin. The same heterogeneity of NAID was seen in both studies, with evidence that the NAID infants in both studies performed at equivalent levels to control infants, and that eventually all nonanemic infants presented no overt developmental derangements.

Lozoff's 52 infants with iron deficiency anemia corresponded to our anemic group. She found differences in MDI and PDI. In PDI, only moderate anemics (< 10 g/dl) were affected, whereas all anemics had low MDI. Her infants with moderate anemia had PDI scores like those of our intermediate group (hemoglobin of 10.5–10.9 g/dl) in the hemoglobin versus development index graph (Fig. 4). With respect to intervening variables, we did not perform HOME (home inventory observation scale) evaluations or determine parental intelligence quotients; however, all of the other evaluated parameters were the same. In any event, these variables did not influence our results or Lozoff's findings, since anemia remained the strongest single determinant of psychomotor performance.

The distribution of the BSID scores of the children in Lozoff's study showed—as did ours—that her selection process had also biased out those children with low performance scores, unlike her previous study in Guatemala. Mean scores in her study were somewhat higher than ours, and motor indices were not lower than mental performances in her infants; if anything, they were perhaps higher. We have no explanation for these findings. The congruence of the patterns of the raw scores in the two studies is impressive. The alterations in the mental items that relate to language and verbal expression, as well as the motor items related to walking and body balance, even in older children where more complex tasks are required, are very consistent (Table 7). The interpretation of MDI scores in the Lozoff study at 3 months of observation is different because of an unexplained drop in the mean MDI score for the nonanemic group. However, an improvement

TABLE 6. *Criteria for classification of iron nutritional status in the Lozoff study*[a]

	Hgb	FEP (µg ZPP/dl)	Sat% (Fe/TIBC)	SF (µg/L)
Anemic	< 10.5	—	—	—
Intermediate	10.6–11.9	—	—	—
Nonanemic	> 12.0	—	—	—
Iron-sufficient	—	≤ 100	> 10	> 12
Iron-depleted	—	≤ 100	> 10	≤ 12
Iron-deficient	—	> 100	≤ 10	≤ 12

[a]Data from ref. 2 by permission of *Pediatrics*, © 1987.

in MDI for those infants with mild anemia who achieved a full hematological correction speaks for a possible recovery of these infants.

Since Lozoff did not report the age of these infants, it is not possible to relate severity of anemia to age. In our study, we did not find improvement in any of the infants after 3 months of iron therapy, even in the nine anemic infants who completely corrected their iron status, but there might be an age component difference in Lozoff's data that could be important. Older infants with mild anemia probably acquired their iron deficiency later, so that physiological derangements might be easier to reverse with therapy, whereas the infants in our study probably acquired their iron deficit at an earlier age. Reversibility of these putative deficits may be related not only to severity of anemia, but also to the age of onset of iron deprivation.

Many of the criticisms raised about both of these studies stem from the poor predictive value of the Bayley Scales of Infant Development. This point is well taken and indisputable. Nevertheless, to date, all studies carried out relating iron status to cognitive and motor development in this age group have used the BSID as the "gold standard" for lack of a better test. Future research must go beyond the use of the BSID, by employing more sensitive psychological tools, such as visual or auditory attention paradigms, and psychophysiological experiments using attention correlates such as heart rate, skin galvanic conductivity, or pupil size. Neurophysiological measures of nerve and synaptic function in the central nervous system, such as brainstem-evoked potentials and sleep–wakefulness cycle studies both in long-term and short-term (nap) situations, may substantiate the neurological substrate of the Bayley Scales of Infant Development findings in iron-deficient infants. Finally, sophisticated neurochemical tools will have to be developed to detect metabolic alterations in the infant brain "in vivo," such as position emission tomography techniques using labeled neurotransmitter precursors.

TABLE 7. *Specific patterns of task failure observed by Lozoff*[a]

Mental Development Index Items
   Showing own shoes
   Placing pegs on pegboard
   Naming one object
Psychomotor Development Index Items
   Walking alone
   Standing up from supine position
   Standing on left foot with help
   Standing up
   Balancing on left foot alone
   Walking up or down stairs

[a]From ref. 2 with permission by *Pediatrics*, © 1987.

REFERENCES

1. Oski, F. A., and Honig, A. S. (1978): The effects of therapy on the developmental scores of iron deficient infants. *J. Pediatr.*, 92:21–25.
2. Lozoff, B., Brittenham, G. M., Wolf, A. W., et al. (1987): Iron deficiency anemia and iron therapy effects on infant developmental test performance. *Pediatrics*, 79:981–995.
3. Walter, T., DeAndraca, I., Chadud, P., and Perales, C. G. (1989): Adverse effect of iron deficiency anemia on infant psycho-motor development. *Pediatrics* (scheduled for publication).
4. Bayley, N. (1969): *Bayley Scales of Infant Developmental Manual.* Psychological Corporation, New York.
5. Kopp, C. B., and McCall, R. B. (1982): Predicting later mental performance for normal at risk, and handicapped infants. *Life-Span Dev. Behav.*, 4:33–61.
6. Lozoff, B., and Brittenham, G. M. (1985): Behavioral aspects of iron deficiency. *Prog. Hematol.*, 14:23–25.
7. Werner, E., and Bayley, N. (1966): The reliability of Bayley's revised scale of mental and motor development during the first year of life. *Child Dev.*, 37:39–50.
8. Siimes, M. A., Refino, C., and Dallman, P. R. (1980): Manifestations of iron deficiency at various levels of dietary iron intake. *Am. J. Clin. Nutr.*, 33:570–574.
9. Leibel, R. L. (1977): Behavioral and biochemical correlates of iron deficiency. *J. Am. Diet Assoc.*, 71:398–422.
10. Walter, T., Kovalskys, J., and Stekel, A. (1983): Effect of mild iron deficiency on infant mental development scores. *J. Pediatr.*, 102:519–522.
11. Matheny, A. P., Jr. (1980): Bayley's infant behavior record: behavioral components and twin analyses. *Child Dev.*, 51:1157–1167.

Dietary Iron: Birth to Two Years,
edited by L. J. Filer, Jr.
Raven Press, Ltd., New York © 1989.

Discussion

Dr. Filer: Did Dr. Lozoff give criteria for her classification of anemia?

Dr. Walter: Dr. Lozoff's classification for anemia differed from ours in that she did not use response to iron therapy as a classification criteria. She had to set her criteria to make sure that her anemic infants were really anemic or had a high probability of being anemic and that her normal infants had a high probability of being iron-sufficient. Also, the community that she studied is located 1,100 m above sea level, so she needed to set her hemoglobin levels slightly above what is expected at sea level.

Dr. Filer: Were the mental development indices of the anemic subjects in Dr. Lozoff's study still considered normal within the population?

Dr. Walter: Yes. However, even if a child is within the normal range, he or she could still function better with a higher hemoglobin.

Dr. Filer: Do you have any data to show that anemia is causing permanent damage in mental and motor function? By suppressing growth, one can delay development or the aging process. This may be occurring in your studies and with time the infants will catch up.

Dr. Walter: Those are good questions and I do not have good answers. Neither Dr. Lozoff nor I has data to answer these questions at the present time. However, I know that the infants in both studies are being evaluated in long-term follow-up studies.

Dr. Ziegler: How can you be sure that the anemic children are not different at the onset of the study?

Dr. Walter: In our study, the only determinant of iron status was the random assignment to the fortification versus the nonfortification group. Consequently, most of the anemic infants were in the non-iron-fortification group. Of course, we performed covariant analyses of the intervening variables and multiple regression analyses. As soon as hemoglobin level or iron status was entered into the analysis, all other differences were erased.

Dr. Dallman: Dr. Walter is the only one who has done a study in which randomization occurred early on so that many of the concerns about the effects of other variables such as the home situation or the education of the mother are not factors.

Dr. Oski: Dr. Walter, since you did not show any effects of iron deficiency in the absence of anemia, how certain are you that it is iron deficiency rather than anemia that is having an effect? Have you studied any children who have anemia for other reasons?

Dr. Walter: No I have not.

Dr. Oski: I was surprised to see that after 3 months of iron therapy, only 10 of 36 children in your study and only 9 of 30 children in Dr. Lozoff's study achieved normal iron status. How do we know it was not something plus the iron that resulted in the failure to improve?

Dr. Walter: Both Dr. Lozoff and I followed all of the infants until their iron status was corrected. We gave them 1 or 2 more months of iron therapy just to make sure that it was iron and nothing else. They were receiving Fer-In-Sol (ferrous sulfate), not a multivitamin–iron preparation.

Dietary Iron: Birth to Two Years,
edited by L. J. Filer, Jr.
Raven Press, Ltd., New York © 1989.

The Interaction of Lead and Iron

Ray Yip

*Division of Nutrition, Center for Chronic Disease Prevention and Health Promotion,
Centers for Disease Control, Atlanta, Georgia 30333*

Childhood lead poisoning and iron deficiency anemia are two major pediatric public health issues. The interactions between lead poisoning and iron deficiency are multiple and strong enough that it may be appropriate to consider that lead poisoning is one of the adverse consequences of iron deficiency. For lead poisoning to occur, two important risk factors must be present. First, there must be exposure to a source of lead, and thus only a subset of iron-deficient individuals is affected. The second necessary risk factor is behavioral. One can live in an environment that is heavily contaminated with lead, but a hand-to-mouth motion must happen fairly frequently for lead poisoning to occur. This behavioral risk factor can also be related to iron deficiency. Iron deficiency may be the strongest nutritional risk factor.

The evidence for a socioeconomic interaction between lead poisoning and iron deficiency anemia is from epidemiological data. A common risk factor for both iron deficiency and lead poisoning is a low socioeconomic background. Poor families living in poor high-lead housing are likely to have poor nutrition. The NHANES II survey data on blood lead levels can be arrayed into the percentages of children who have elevated blood lead levels in five income and five educational level groupings. That analysis shows that the prevalence of elevated blood lead levels is highest in the less educated or lower-income families. The prevalence of iron deficiency anemia follows a similar gradient across the socioeconomic spectrum. These data do not necessarily mean that there is a causal relationship, but they do show that the risks tend to occur in persons who are at the lower end of the spectrum for education or income.

The clinical evidence comes from several studies that show that lead exposure is greater in children who are iron-deficient than in those who are not iron deficient. In addition, children with increased lead absorption are more likely to be iron-deficient. In a study of 43 children living in Minneapolis who fit the CDC criteria for lead poisoning (i.e., blood lead levels greater than 30 µg/dl and protoporphyrin levels that ranged from 35 to 50 µg/dl), we classified 29 children as having mild lead poisoning and 14 children with moderate lead poisoning. Iron deficiency was defined by low transferrin saturation and low blood ferritin values. The prevalence of iron deficiency was 79% in the mild lead poisoning group and 100% in the moderate lead poisoning group (Table 1). The iron-deficiency rate in our baseline population was 10%. The prevalence of anemia in the mild and moderate lead poisoning groups was 24% and 43%, respectively. If we divide the NHANES II data for children 1 to 12 years of age into groups according to transferrin saturation, we find that children with the lowest transferrin saturation are three times as likely to have elevated lead levels as the children whose transferrin saturation is greater than 30% (Table 2). If the data are adjusted for age, the differences are not as dramatic but the relationship is the same.

The behavioral interaction is related to the fact that pica or the hand-to-mouth motion is a very important causative factor of childhood lead poisoning in contaminated households. There are a number of reports that suggest that iron-deficient children are more likely to have pica. There are also reports from the adult literature that some bizarre food habits are correctable with iron treatment. Perhaps iron deficiency results in an increase in this particular type of behavior.

Protoporphyrin levels are used to screen for lead toxicity and iron deficiency. The anemia of lead poisoning is commonly regarded as a manifestation of the lead poisoning; however, if one checks the iron nutritional status, very few lead poisoning cases actually have anemia without iron deficiency. Therefore, many of the commonly reported cases of lead poison-

TABLE 1. *Iron nutritional status of children with increased lead absorption (Minneapolis)**

Pb poisoning	Number	Iron deficiency	Anemia
Mild	29	79%	24%
Moderate	14	100%	43%
All	43	86%	30%

*From Yip R, Norris TN, Anderson AS. Iron status of children with elevated blood lead concentrations. *Journal of Pediatrics* 1981;98:922–925.

TABLE 2. *Association of iron deficiency and elevated blood lead in children 1–12 years of age, NHANES II, 1976–1980**

Fe/TIBC (%)	Percentage with Pb > 30 μg/dl
< 10	3.4%
10–30	2.2%
> 30	1.1%

*Centers for Disease Control. *Preventing lead poisoning in young children.* Centers for Disease Control, Atlanta, 1985.

ing anemia can be attributed to iron deficiency. Protoporphyrin values should be regarded as the composite result of both lead and iron status. In NHANES II, the individuals with the most elevated protoporphyrin levels were the ones with the highest lead levels and lowest iron levels.

The evidence for a physiological interaction between lead and iron comes from a series of animal experiments showing that lead absorption is significantly increased in iron-deficient animals. Also, human studies using radioisotopes of lead indicate that iron-deficient individuals absorb more lead than normal individuals. There is additional evidence from animal studies that shows that there is increased tissue retention of lead in iron-deficient states.

All of this evidence suggests that these interactions may be more than just coincidence and that there may be a cause-and-effect relationship. Therefore, childhood lead poisoning might be considered one of the adverse consequences of iron deficiency.

Dietary Iron: Birth to Two Years,
edited by L. J. Filer, Jr.
Raven Press, Ltd., New York © 1989.

Final Comments

Frank A. Oski

*Department of Pediatrics, Johns Hopkins University School of Medicine,
Baltimore, Maryland 21205*

In children under 2 years of age, iron stores and iron intake have to be equivalent or greater than the need for iron for growth and due to losses. An inadequate iron intake is the primary cause of iron deficiency. This is due to either early introduction of cow's milk or the feeding of non-iron-fortified formula. The second leading cause of iron deficiency is the high rate of growth relative to iron endowment at birth and dietary intake of iron. This occurs primarily in preterm infants who become iron-deficient not because they are not getting iron but because their daily dietary intake of iron can not keep up with their rate of growth. A much less common cause of iron deficiency is impaired iron absorption that occurs because the iron used to fortify infant foods is not bioavailable or because the infant is being fed an unusual diet, one very high in protein or inadequate in vitamin C, or the infant is consuming tea or other foods that block iron absorption. Chronic recurrent illnesses may impair iron absorption but that is a very unusual cause of iron deficiency in the U.S. Finally, a child may have decreased iron absorption if there is a gastrointestinal illness that causes bleeding or if the child has polyps. Most iron deficiency in infants and children in the U.S. is due to dietary factors; other causes are much less common.

SUBJECT INDEX

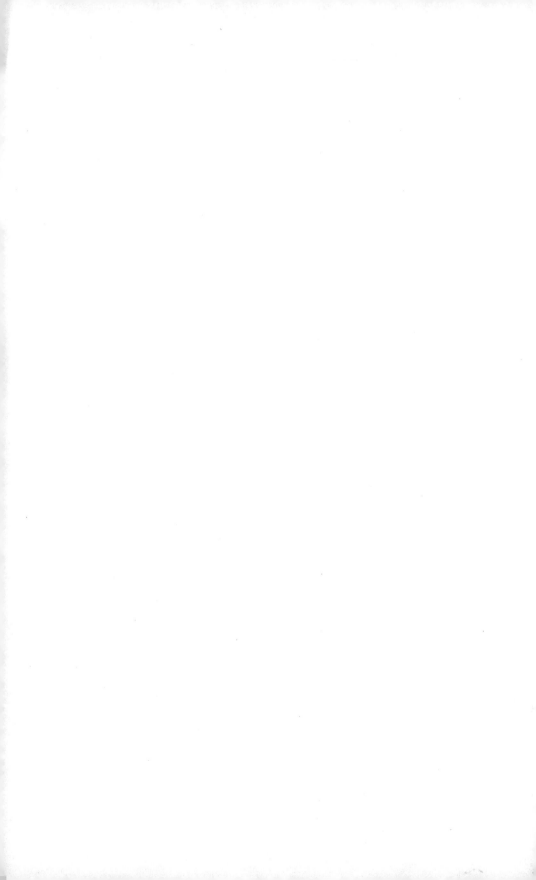